GO TO SLEEP LATE

and other advice for **NIGHT OWLS**

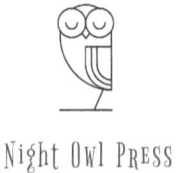

Night Owl Press

Sylvia Dziuba

First published in 2023

Copyright © 2023 by Sylvia Dziuba

All rights reserved.

No portion of this book may be reproduced in any form or by any means, electronic or mechanical, including photocopying, recording or by any other information storage and retrieval system, without prior written permission from the publisher or author.

The Australian Copyright Act 1968 (the Act) allows a maximum of one chapter or 10 per cent of the book, whichever is greater, to be photocopied by an educational institution for its educational purposes, provided that the educational institution (or body that administers it) has given a remuneration notice to the Copyright Agency (Australia) under the Act.

Night Owl Press
Salisbury North SA 5108
email: hello@sylviadziuba.com

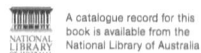
A catalogue record for this book is available from the National Library of Australia

ISBN 978-0-6455412-0-5

For my husband Greg, who has always
loved and supported me

Contents

1. How It All Started   1
   - Note
   - Disclaimer

2. Rhythm   11
   - What is circadian rhythm?
   - A little bit of history
   - What is circadian misalignment?
   - Is the circadian rhythm flexible?
   - What happens when our rhythm is disrupted?
   - Some stats & facts

3. Chronotype   33
   - Are you a biological night owl?
   - How are night owls different?
   - Night owls at different stages of life
   - Can night owls become early larks?

    A word to the sceptic

4. Body   56
    Your master clock predicts the future
    The anatomy of sleep
    Insomnia and early death
    Female-specific issues
    Male-specific issues

5. Mind   70
    Living in an early-riser society
    Neurological deterioration
    Cognitive impairment

6. Work   77
    Career
    Physical work
    Cognitive work
    Athletes
    Entrepreneurs

7. Parenting   92
    Newborns and young children
    Adolescents

8. Life   103

    Appointments
    Going out
    Attitudes
    Exercise
    Study
    Eating
    Naps
    Biphasic sleep
    Environment
    Meditation
    Travel
    Illness

9. Conclusion — 126

About the Author — 129

Acknowledgements — 131

Chapter One

How It All Started

For many years I heard, read and – gasp! – believed the well-intentioned advice of the early risers, the ones who just cannot wait to jump out of bed at 5 am and put on their running shoes. You can often hear these early birds in the wee hours of the morning, singing their little hearts out in the shower.

The advice can be best summed up as: wake up early, exercise, eat your breakfast, and you'll be healthy and wealthy forever and ever, amen. But I did believe this 'good' advice and tried my best to apply it in my own life – can you blame me? I, too, wanted to be successful, because this is what successful people do. Right?

The people that eagerly spread these 'facts' tend to reference books such as *The 7 Habits of Highly Effective People* and use social media to post slogans such as 'The first step to winning is to wake up early', often eloquently backed up with science, quoting study after study to validate these exclamations of 'truth'.

Do they ever consider that what is true for them may not be true for everyone? We are **not** all created alike!

Some of us are right-handed, others are lefties, some of us revel in a humid summer's day, others prefer the cold, some have an allergic reaction to peanuts, others can eat bucketloads of the stuff. Do you see where I'm going with this?

Our biology differs from person to person, and trying to give good advice by throwing everyone into a single bucket is not only unwise but outright dangerous. This is especially true when saying that everyone should wake up early.

To illustrate my point, I'd like to offer the example of right-handers vs. left-handers. History has shown how the majority – the right-handers – tried to force the lefties to be just like them, convinced that the right hand is the most effective, fastest and only appropriate way to write. They tried to force left-handers to change, to fit in with society; if they refused, the lefties were punished, ridiculed and treated like lesser human beings.

Thankfully, we don't do that anymore. We now understand that, in most cases, when using their right hand, a lefty will never be able to write as well, as aesthetically pleasing or as fast as they would with their left hand, regardless of how hard they push themselves or how often they practise. Why can't we adopt the same attitude towards night owls?

Having said that, I realise night owls are not the majority – according to statistics, night owls represent only about 20% of the population – which is a good thing because, overall, society functions best when most people rise in the morning. But that same society needs night owls – the security guards, nurses, doctors, firefighters etc. – those who work while others sleep.

In my case, I continued to push myself to fit into this 'socially acceptable' lifestyle, to make sure I was perceived as a responsible adult and respectable member of society. I had no other choice. Working as a project manager in the construction sector meant early mornings and long days.

This was not conducive to my late-phase chronotype (a scientific term for a night owl), yet I persevered, dragging myself out of bed after yet another measly four to five hours of sleep. Trying my best to pretend I was awake while looking at the world through a thick fog – I'd force every cell in my body to press on.

Sometimes it all got too much, and instead of eating lunch like a normal, well-behaved employee, I would sleep in my car.

Every now and again, I'd hear people talk about the night-owl syndrome, but mostly as a joke or a myth used primarily with negative undertones. Often, the term is associated with irresponsible, party-going teenagers or people that are lazy or those living with a mental illness or substance abuse – I wasn't ready to join that crowd.

Even some of my family and closest friends told me that my 'sleeping problem' was all in my head, that all I needed was to change some of my habits and get my act together – otherwise, I'd end up ruining my life. This well-intentioned advice further fuelled my internal monologue of what a crap human being I was.

The thing is, no matter how many consecutive mornings I'd spend waking up at exactly 6 am, or what else I did – exposing myself to morning sun; not taking a nap during the day; following the experts' advice to slowly ease into a bedtime routine by not watching TV; turning off my phone and reading a book by warm dim light; making sure that my linen was all-natural and that the bedroom temperature was 'just right'; and going to bed at the same time each night at 10:30 pm – I'd still be lying there, wide awake at 2 am, every single night!

When I couldn't handle any more self-criticism, I looked to shift the blame elsewhere; that's when I started to wonder whether I was suffering from insomnia.

By then, I was well into my forties and going to sleep was a nightmare (pun intended) associated with plenty of discomfort, tossing and pain – physical and emotional. Then came Covid, restrictions and lockdowns – I lost my job. This was a blessing in disguise because it was around this time that I was at my wit's end. I thought, 'Enough is enough!' I can't live like a zombie anymore: forever longing for the weekend to sleep off my nightly deficit.

So, while the never-ending pandemic lockdowns were in effect, I decided to run an experiment. I promised that I would no longer go to bed unless I genuinely felt sleepy, regardless of what time it was.

At that point, I decided to take my writing seriously and pursue a passion I'd had all my life.

However, while running the experiment, I also promised myself that in addition to waking up naturally – no alarm clock – and going to sleep when sleepy, I would only work when my brain felt awake and productive.

For the first time in my life, my 'insomnia' was gone, and I actually fell asleep within minutes of going to bed – this was heaven!

Is this what life could be like? Not only did I feel rested, clear and in a good mood upon waking, I didn't have to force myself to do anything. I was able to easily process information – I felt happy! My body felt good, my mind felt good – I was productive like never before!

Originally, I thought I was going to run this experiment for a month. Little did I know the experiment would never end. The whole experience left me feeling so good, emotionally and physically, that I lost some unwanted weight – which, until that point, had been steadily climbing over the years.

Most importantly, I knew that I would never go back to my previous job, not that I didn't enjoy it, I did, but I realised that continuing on that path was no longer in the best interest of my emotional or physical health.

At that point, writing was still a side hustle, a hobby that I enjoyed doing freelance – after hours, outside of my day job. This seemed like a perfect opportunity to take my writing seriously.

In my case, the career switch wasn't hard as I love writing. It was more the psychological switch to rely financially on a somewhat unsteady income source. But I put all my energy into it and managed to get a few regular freelance writing gigs. I also enrolled at university to get a degree in writing and publishing (thank you, Curtin University).

So, what does my routine look like today?

I normally go to sleep around 2 am, then wake up naturally around 7 to 8 hours later – without an alarm clock. My experiment has now turned into a permanent lifestyle choice; I no longer struggle to fall or stay asleep. I'm able to stay productive and alert – and happy – all day long. Well, for full disclosure, I do nap – sometimes.

My personal experience has triggered an urge to help others. But in order to do so, I needed to find out what science has to say about this. So, I dove headfirst into all the research I could find about sleeping and chronobiology (the study of circadian rhythms).

What I discovered blew my mind. It was the best thing I could do to alleviate any remaining feelings of guilt about my new routine. I wrote this book to share all that I learned – I hope you'll find the contents as helpful and freeing as I did.

Even though this book starts off anecdotally, it isn't based on my personal experience but rather on thorough scientific research. In preparation, I read a multitude of books, research papers, studies and literature reviews by top scientists and experts in this field; they are listed in the acknowledgements section, at the end of this book.

Note

In the process of reading all the aforementioned studies, research papers, books, articles, expert opinions etc., I was forced to learn a slew of scientific jargon – in order to understand what I was researching.

I'd like to spare you the torture of that experience, so I've written this book in its simplest form. This means that I use basic words and metaphors to try and explain some of the complex concepts I came across in my research. For example, I use the terms **clock** or **master clock** instead of ***suprachiasmatic nuclei*** – its scientific term – to refer to the timekeeper located in your brain. I hope you appreciate that :)

I also wanted you to be able to read freely, without distractions, so I decided to keep it free of footnotes pointing to the studies and research I'm quoting.

However, for those of you who are more curious, I've compiled a detailed reference list that includes all the sources on which this book was based.

You can find this on my website:

https://sylviadziuba.com/go-to-sleep-late/research/

Disclaimer

Please understand that your body is a unique and complex organism, and what has worked for me might not work for you. As such, the advice in this book does not constitute medical advice, and I highly recommend you first consult a doctor or a specialist about your unique situation before making any radical changes to your lifestyle.

Chapter Two

Rhythm

What is circadian rhythm?

Living in today's society, most people have some idea about the inherent link between sleep, health and cognition. According to leading researcher David Samson, sleep plays a critical role in regulating our immune system, memory retention, focus, decision-making and physical performance.

But it goes far beyond that. Because it isn't just how long you sleep that matters; science is increasingly discovering that an even more important factor that determines the quality of your sleep – and its related benefits – is **when you sleep**.

The fact is that everybody has a 24-hour master clock. Everyone has an ideal time for sleeping, eating and performing physical and cognitive tasks. Functioning outside that framework carries serious consequences – as discussed in subsequent chapters.

Your master clock is composed of 20,000 to 50,000 neurons and goes by the scientific name of 'suprachiasmatic nuclei' or SCN for short. It sits inside the hypothalamus – in the middle of your brain, just behind the roof of your mouth.

The master clock controls your 24-hour cycle – a sequence of biological events that fire in specific order. Your brain, every organ, the microbiome and each cell in your body marches to the drum of your master clock.

This book focuses on the four most important aspects of that 24-hour cycle:

1. sleeping,

2. eating,

3. cognition,

4. physical activity.

> Note: The next few paragraphs are going to get a little more technical, but I ask you to bear with me as they are fundamental to the rest of the book.

The 24-hour circadian cycle occurs irrespective of where you are and what you do. It means that even if you were left in a dark room without any windows for weeks or months on end, your body would still follow the same daily routine by making you feel awake/sleepy almost at the same time each day. I say 'almost' because most people's cycles are not exactly 24 hours, and the master clock depends on external signals, such as light, to 'adjust' and keep itself on time.

This daily adjustment relies on a specialised blue-light sensing protein called 'melanopsin' – produced by cells found in your retina called the *ganglion cells* – discovered by three separate labs between 1999 and 2002.

The melanopsin protein is present in about 5,000 neurons (in each eye) and hardwired to the master clock. What's interesting is that people with impaired vision also rely on this protein; even when the person's vision is severely impaired or completely gone, as long as they have eyes, these cells remain unencumbered and are able to 'see and read' the light. The colour and tone of the light allow them to identify what time of day it is and communicate that to the master clock. Light cues are vital in helping to maintain or readjust our circadian rhythm; if we didn't have them, we wouldn't be able to function properly when changing time zones or navigating seasonal changes.

***

The 24-hour rhythm refers to the term 'circadian', which is derived from Latin *circa diem*, meaning about a day. This means that the clock is rarely exactly 24 hours. For some people, that clock operates on just under 24 hours, defined as an 'advanced cycle', which is usually characteristic of morning larks.

However, most people's clocks – including night owls – are slightly longer than 24 hours (approximately 24.2 hours), which is why we need light to adjust our rhythm on a daily basis. In the case of extreme night owls – the ones that go to sleep veeery late – some evidence suggests that their cycles might be even longer than the average 24.2 hours.

Your daily sleep–wake cycle (the circadian rhythm) is controlled by two primary drivers: the **master clock** and **sleep pressure**.

The first driver, the master clock, controls and synchronises many other clocks in your body, larger and smaller, down to the cellular level, with each cell having its own 24-hour clock. These clocks operate on a continuous conversation loop with the master clock, sending and receiving information that is 'read and evaluated' by the clock. The clock uses this information to plan and adjust all biological processes, optimising sequences according to your body's needs.

The second driver, sleep pressure, is a chemical substance called 'adenosine' that slowly builds up in your body over the span of the day. Its job is to make you feel relaxed and sleepy.

It is the influence of these two drivers that directly affect how tired or alert you feel at any given time during the 24-hour cycle.

A little bit of history

This section gives you a deeper look at the major milestones in chronobiology research, but if you find it 'too much', go to the end of this section, where I've provided an easy-to-read summary. However, if you are like me and find the little details fascinating, by all means, jump right in.

The study of chronobiology originated in the 18th century. However, for the longest time, the research was fairly rudimentary and primarily focused on plants and animals.

The first recorded study was by a French astronomer Jean-Jacques d'Ortous de Mairan who discovered that the leaves of the heliotrope plant opened and closed at the same time during a 24-hour cycle, even when it was kept in complete darkness.

Subsequently, similar experiments were carried out on other plants, animals, then finally, humans.

The first study carried out on humans was undertaken in a cave, then in an underground bunker, in complete darkness. Both proved that, like most plants and animals, we also have a 24-hour cycle.

In the 1960s, Patricia DeCoursey discovered the relationship between light signals and mammals' circadian rhythm and invented the *phase response curve*. Her research is still used today to expand our understanding of light and its role in resetting/disrupting our biological clocks. We can see this research implemented into our daily lives. For example, the night-shift function on your devices, which changes the display colour and brightness on our phones and computers helps to reduce circadian rhythm disruptions.

In the 1970s, Franz Halberg coined the term 'circadian', but much to his disappointment – since he was keen to see more human studies – most of the chronobiology research in the '70s was still primarily focused on animals and plants. It was during this time that the protagonist of our story, the master clock or suprachiasmatic nuclei, was discovered – in 1972, to be exact.

Nonetheless, most of human chronobiology research is relatively new. It wasn't until the early 2000s that a couple of major breakthroughs in human studies took place. One was the discovery of the aforementioned melanopsin – the photoreceptor protein inside the ganglion cells located in your retina. It was during this period that scientists also discovered the link between clock genes and human diseases, including cancer. In 2004–05, scientists established the link between clock disruption and impaired metabolism. And in 2014–15, the master clock's control of the immune system was confirmed.

In 2016, a genome-wide association study was conducted, where scientists began identifying specific genes responsible for our circadian rhythm. At first, they discovered nine gene sets; then, in 2018, this number grew to 24. But the most significant chronobiology study took place in 2019, when the scientific world discovered a total of – wait for it – 351 gene sets directly connected to chronotypes! This was a huge breakthrough; the study analysed almost 700,000 individuals and revealed many interesting facts about our sleeping preferences. It also established strong links between depression and disrupted circadian rhythm – particularly pertaining to night owls. You can read the paper in the *Nature Communications* journal.

In simple terms, the studies confirmed what many instinctively knew all along: it's hardwired genes that cause a morning person to wake up early, all happy, full of energy and mentally alert, while waking up a night owl early in the morning just makes them angry.

It isn't that our modern society wasn't innately aware of the differences between people's preferred sleeping styles prior to these findings; it's just that modern society has attached a stigma to those favouring a delayed rhythm. However, this wasn't always the case.

For example, some historians claim that during medieval times, teenage boys – who are all, temporarily, night owls – were intentionally selected to keep night-watch on city walls to protect its inhabitants at night; because it was evident that they didn't need much willpower to stay awake until the wee hours of the morning.

Also, day naps were customary throughout history and formed part of standard daily routine. We know this not just from books and biographies but from testimonies found in court transcripts dating back to the Middle Ages. In fact, when I lived in Greece – back in 1988 – my sister and I almost got arrested for playing ball outside during siesta. I'm not quite sure what it's like today, but back then, all shops closed, and all trades stopped in the middle of the day for about 2 to 3 hours, for a customary nap.

While some cultures may still practice the afternoon siesta today, for most Western societies, it was during the industrial era that evening types (and nappers) began to be increasingly perceived as lazy and irresponsible.

The Western culture and the desire for homogeneity have deprived us of common sense and practical thinking. We became blind to the utility of night owls, disregarding the benefits this natural state offers society. We started looking at night owls as less-than: a group of people that needed to be fixed. Even today, many scientists still refer to the late-phase syndrome as a 'late-phase **disorder**' – yikes!

Overall, chronobiology research has exploded in the last two decades, with hundreds of studies and research papers in the field of general medicine as well as psychology. The findings have increased our understanding of biological rhythms, aided the development of many inventions and increased public awareness that, in the end, help us all to live healthier and longer lives.

Section summary: The study of chronobiology began in the 18th century; however, until recently, most studies were animal and plant oriented. The most notable human-centred studies began around the year 2000, with the most significant discoveries taking place between 2014 and 2019.

The most important findings were associated with the links between the clock and the immune system, metabolism and psychology – and the vital role of light in aligning the circadian clock.

Seeing that most of these findings have only come to light in recent years, we should be more understanding when people are a little sceptical when you tell them that you're a genetic night owl. The scientific data is still fairly new and hasn't spread widely enough to the general population.

What is circadian misalignment?

The term *social jetlag* – coined by Dr Till Roenneberg from Ludwig Maximilian University in Munich – describes the repeated mismatch between a person's circadian rhythm and their work and education demands, causing chronic sleep deprivation. This is particularly true for night owls.

It's what happens to you when you wake up early in the morning, forcing your circadian rhythm out of whack – every single day! It feels like you're continually jet-lagged, living in a different time zone and carries long-term consequences for your physical and mental health.

Circadian misalignment happens when you ask your body to do something at the wrong time; to perform a task, the body hasn't planned for that particular stage of the 24-hr cycle. For example, if I woke you up in the middle of the night from your deepest sleep and immediately started asking you complicated algebra questions, even if you were actually good at maths and genuinely tried to help me (as opposed to biting my head off, which would be a more natural response). No matter how hard you tried, your answers would most likely be delayed or even inaccurate. It's also scientifically proven that if you tried to drive your car at this point (with only a few hours of sleep), your performance would be worse than if you were legally drunk.

Your biology works on a highly orchestrated sequence of events. Every cell in your body has its own routine. It goes through cycles of active, resting and restorative periods. And each one of those is orchestrated in alignment with other cells' cycles, all connecting to larger and more sophisticated systems and functions in the body.

Is the circadian rhythm flexible?

Even though our circadian rhythm is controlled by the master clock, dictating our optimum sleeping-eating-active time, limited research suggests that some people's clocks are more flexible than others.

What this means in practice is that some people are able to push their sleep–wake times slightly backwards or forwards while still maintaining a high level of cognitive and physical competence. This is usually limited to anywhere from 30 minutes to a couple of hours, depending on each person's unique biology. However, it can only be achieved by a change in eating and activity habits, and, most importantly, by well-timed exposure to sunlight – or sun-mimicking light.

In a 2019 study led by chronobiology and performance expert Dr Elise Facer-Childs, 21 participants – all night owls – were able to adjust their rhythm back by two hours.

However, after a brief follow-up, it was found that some of them reverted back to their original sleep–wake cycles.

However, the majority of scientists involved in this field are not convinced the clock is flexible. Matthew Walker PhD, a neuroscientist, researcher and the world's leading sleep expert, suggests that each person's circadian rhythm is genetically fixed and can only be minimally adjusted by about 30 to 45 minutes either way. The only way to push it further is through a change in time zones or when we experience the change of seasons – through external cues, primarily the light–dark cycles synchronising our master clock.

Based on my own experience, I tend to side with Walker. There is far more research that proves our clocks are uncompromising, meaning that no matter what you do – short of flying to another time zone – your body will stick to a solid regimen of lowering your eyelids and waking you up at a similar time each day, to the point where sometimes you wake up at the same time each day, regardless of how much sleep you had the night before. It's almost as if your master clock is saying, 'Good morning, we've got work to do; it's time to start the day.'

I also think that if you are able to successfully wake up two hours earlier every day than you used to, you were probably off your circadian rhythm to begin with, and the new regimen has reset your clock in alignment with your true genetic chronotype.

I am not the only one who believes that changing your circadian rhythm, even with the best of intentions, is impossible. Well-known author Brandon Sanderson is a self-proclaimed night owl, who usually goes to sleep around 4 am. But when he got married, his wife – a morning lark – begged him to change his ways so that they could go to bed together, which would make their life much easier. Being young and in love, he tried to switch with all the willpower he could muster. Finally, after yet another torturous night of lying in bed completely awake and not being to function during the day, his wife couldn't watch him suffer any more and agreed that he should go back to his night-owl routine, for the sake of both their sanity.

> A 2016 paper in the Journal of Chronobiology International concludes that, in some cases, marital problems may be caused by the

couple's mismatched chronotypes and proposes sleeping apart as a possible solution.

But I hear you say, 'Of course, he can afford to go to sleep at 4 am – he's a writer. He doesn't have a day job like the rest of us.' Well, you might be surprised to discover that there are plenty of night owls with a day job. One of the best examples is the co-founder of Reddit, Alexis Ohanian, who says that he never goes to bed before 3 am. He normally wakes up after 10:00 am, yet manages to run a multi-million-dollar business that continues to thrive.

Bryan Clayton, the CEO of GreenPal gets out of bed around 9 am. He tried waking up at 5 am with his previous jobs but says that 'After forcing myself for over six months to crack dawn every morning, I realised that I was half as effective as I was when I was getting 8 to 9 hours of sleep every day'.

Although these are examples of people high up in the corporate hierarchy, there are many examples of everyday people, working standard jobs, who have successfully negotiated alternative starting–finishing hours with their employers to accommodate their nightly routine.

This is particularly prevalent in Denmark, where B-Society (an organisation that advocates for chronotype equality) works with businesses of all sizes, including government agencies, to negotiate working hours for night owls in both white-collar and blue-collar jobs.

What happens when our rhythm is disrupted?

As mentioned earlier, an average person's natural body cycle is about 24.2 hours long. If left to run its course, your natural body clock would shift your sleep-wake pattern an hour forward every 5 days, ultimately pushing you into misalignment with any social or professional routines. This is why the master clock needs light, especially the natural dawn and dusk light, to help it synchronise with a solar day, as per local time zone or season.

Even though light is the most significant influencer of the master clock, the clock also uses 2 other main drivers to help it synchronise your cycle: consumption and activity. **When** and **what** you eat and **when** you expend the most energy have a huge influence on the consistency of your rhythm.

In addition to these 3 main influencers, the clock 'considers and evaluates' many other external and internal factors, which can be as simple as when you receive a vaccine jab, get upset or happy, or experience physical injury.

These external and internal influencers, combined with the ongoing conversation loop between the master clock and other clocks in the body, allow the master clock to decide when to turn on or off certain biological functions (genes) throughout the day. These functions include sleep, metabolism, memory retention, healing, the release of hormones, and countless others.

The clock's job isn't just to synchronise but to plan ahead and anticipate what your body will require at different times of the day; it plans what to do and when. We disrupt the circadian rhythm when we mess with that plan.

For example, when we cut back on sleep, our prefrontal cortex refuses to go to work. Your prefrontal cortex is the rational centre of your brain; it helps you to, for example, regulate your emotions by keeping calm in the face of provocation. This part of the brain always reminds me of the animated movie *Inside Out* and its command centre, where the emotions, played by eccentric characters, are trying to help Riley navigate her emotional reality.

This should explain why you become a raging lunatic for no apparent reason – or with very little provocation – when you're short on sleep. Have you ever said, 'I wasn't thinking'? Well, you were not – literally; you were trying to reach your prefrontal cortex outside of office hours, and the sign on the door said, 'Access denied'.

Another example of circadian disruption is eating at the wrong time. You might think that a late-night snack or a sip of leftover wine before bed is not a big deal, but do this often enough, and you'll develop some form of metabolic syndrome.

Metabolic syndrome (or metabolic dysfunction) is a cluster of conditions consisting of increased risk of stroke, heart disease, type 2 diabetes and others. These are usually linked to high blood pressure, high cholesterol and blood sugar, and excess fat around the waist. Metabolic disorders can lead to a myriad of other scary conditions, such as Krabbe disease, Hunter syndrome, Gaucher disease and metachromatic leukodystrophy, and many others.

Dr Caroline Sutton, a researcher at Trinity College in Dublin, and her colleagues found in 2017 that continuous disruption of the circadian rhythm also leads to an increased risk of autoimmune disease: a malfunctioning immune system that attacks healthy cells. They found that autoimmune disease is caused by an inflammatory environment in the central nervous system caused by the stress created by prolonged misalignment between a person's lifestyle and their natural body clock. This adds an additional layer of adverse impact on the overall immune system and its ability to respond to the sheer number of attacks it deals with on a daily basis.

***

To round up this section, I want to mention that there is a tiny percentage of the population affected by what is called a *non-24-hour disorder*. This describes a circadian rhythm of 25 (or more) hours, meaning that the person afected by this condition goes to sleep an hour or so later every day. This is extremely rare and mostly affects individuals that have lost their eyes. But if you suspect that you might belong to this group, I highly recommend that you seek the advice of a sleep specialist. However, I will not be covering this disorder here, as the sole object of this book is advice for night owls.

Some stats & facts

RAND, a non-profit research organisation that helps improve policy and decision-making through research and analysis, has conducted research indicating that school and work currently start too early, which has negative consequences on both individuals and the economy.

According to RAND's research, the negative effects of starting school and work too early include decreased performance, diminished academic achievement, increased absenteeism, higher risk of car accidents and workplace accidents, and negative impact on mental and physical health. These effects can be particularly pronounced for adolescents and young adults, who require more sleep than adults – see section on Parenting in Chapter 7.

In terms of the economic cost, RAND estimates that this is costing the US economy around $9 billion annually. This cost is primarily due to decreased productivity and performance, as well as increased healthcare costs associated with the negative health effects of sleep deprivation.

Fatigue-related accidents cause one fatal accident per hour in the United States. And in the UK, statistics show that 57% of junior doctors have either had a crash or a near accident on the drive home after finishing a night shift.

Global studies show that the average divorce rate for night-shift workers is six times higher than for those working day shifts. Considering that only about 20% of the population are night owls, this makes sense – most night-shift workers are either morning larks or intermediates and are functioning out of alignment with their biological cycle.

Cancer patients who align their lifestyle with their circadian system can not only extend their life expectancy but, overall, have a 70% survival rate as opposed to those living in circadian misalignment or constant sleep deprivation, who only have a 40% survival rate.

Chapter Three

Chronotype

Are you a biological night owl?

Figuring out your chronotype is vital for your emotional and physical well-being. Knowing which group you belong to allows you to make informed decisions about your body. It also helps you to better plan your life, from basic everyday tasks like when to eat and exercise to your long-term personal, family and professional/career plans.

Unlike other species that can be classified as either nocturnal or diurnal, humans can belong to more than one type. Science calls these 'chronotypes'. Even though some experts like to use up to 6 categories, for simplicity's sake, most researchers typically divide people into 3 chronotypes: **morning**, **intermediate** and **evening**. The truth is that each person's cycle is unique, but the chronotype distinctions allow researchers to group individuals with 'similar' timing and traits.

It's estimated that around 80% of people belong to the day-dweller camp, which includes the morning larks (about 30% of the population) and the intermediates (50% of the population).

The exact percentage of night owls is hard to estimate because it depends on which scientist you ask. For the most part, it varies from 8% to 30%. Most studies and research papers that I read averaged around the 20% mark, which – for the purposes of this book – is what I'll use when referring to statistics from here on.

***

There are several medical terms for night owls; this includes *delayed sleep phase syndrome* or *delayed sleep–wake phase disorder*; however, many scientists refer to it as simply, *late chronotype*. In Denmark – and other countries – night owls are referred to as *B-persons* (and larks as *A-persons*). There are other terms, but in the end, all of them refer to a group of individuals with delayed biological rhythms, whose genetic makeup differs from the norm.

> Night owls are also known as 'nyctophiles'. According to the Cambridge Dictionary, a nyctophile is someone who is very content and comfortable in the dark – staying up alone late at night, wide awake.

So, how can you tell if you belong to camp nyctophile? Let's start with the obvious signs. The first thing to look for is to notice when your brain is most awake. Night owls find it easiest to maintain a state of sustained focus, mental clarity and creativity at night. And, for the most part, it doesn't even matter whether they feel rested or tired at the time; their brain just goes into overdrive at night and, for some, well into the wee hours of the morning.

Another sign is what happens when your alarm clock goes off early in the morning. If you often greet the morning feeling jetlagged, foggy and ready to kill anyone who dares to take away your coffee, there's a good chance that you might be a biological night owl.

Also, being a late chronotype is genetic – i.e., it is inherited – meaning that if one of your parents or grandparents is a night owl, it increases the chances of you being one as well.

For more scientific proof, get yourself tested at a sleep clinic where they can check what time your body typically releases melatonin, a hormone produced by the pineal gland. Normally, your body will start to release melatonin about 1 to 1 ½ hours before you are due to fall asleep; for night owls, this happens anywhere between the hours of 10:30 pm to 2:00 am, or later.

Lastly, you can track your temperature over several days (best done when you're not sleep-deprived). On average, daily core temperature patterns of a night owl are delayed by 2.5-3 hours in comparison to a day dweller. Normally, your core body temperature begins to drop around 2 hours before bedtime. However, body temperature is not the most reliable indicator, since it can fluctuate depending on many factors such as ovulation (for women), physical activity, environmental factors and immune system response.

If what I've described above sounds like you, you may be hardwired to go to sleep later than the general population. This is pure genetics, something we are born with, like being left or right-handed.

The bad news is that, if you are a night owl, there's nothing you can do to change your inclination to favour – and thrive in – a late rhythm. No amount of caffeine or lack thereof, exposure to light in the early morning, dimming your lights in the evening, or a slow night routine will change that.

Having said all that, there's a chance that your routine is currently out of alignment with your clock. You might have successfully convinced yourself that you're a night owl, but in reality, you might be one of the intermediates whose clock is slightly skewed towards an evening rhythm. However, with a proper reset, you might be able to shift your lifestyle to a slightly earlier time.

***

Even though we each have a unique rhythm, there are factors that can disrupt your 24-hour cycle. Besides your job, the biggest cause of circadian rhythm disruption is food consumption, particularly the type of food and when it is eaten. For example, a study led by researcher Hans Reinke from the University of Duesseldorf in Germany found that eating a high-fat diet will disrupt your circadian rhythm; it will also inform your behaviour by 'instructing' you to eat often, evenly spread out throughout the day, which in turn reinforces the circadian-misalignment loop.

What's important to note is that some night owls are able to fall asleep much earlier than their biological clock due to an overall sleep deficit and the build-up of sleep pressure (adenosine) in their system. This is usually caused by their lifestyle (e.g. having a normal day job) and their ability, or strong willpower, to refrain from napping during the day.

This can be very misleading, making you think that you might actually be a day person. But even though you manage to fall asleep at a socially acceptable hour, your body is technically still awake because the underlying active-phase biological processes continue to function as though you were awake, particularly during the early stages of your 'sleep'. I used apostrophes because this type of sleep is not of the same quality as it would be if you slept in alignment with your circadian rhythm. The easiest way to tell if you fall into this category is to observe how you feel when you wake up to the alarm clock: do you find it hard to awake? Are you feeling tired, groggy and jetlagged? Not just for a few minutes or an hour after you've awoken, but for several hours. Also, if it wasn't for the alarm, would you continue to sleep? For how long?

When a night owl wakes up earlier than the clock anticipated, the body is still in a rest (sleep) phase. So, in order to correct the misalignment, the clock over-activates the stress axis to allow you to function at a basic level. This is why you're unable to reach peak performance until hours later when your active phase kicks in.

However, waking up groggy might also be a sign of other problems, such as sleep apnoea, or it could be as simple as having experienced fragmented sleep caused by incorrect temperature in your bedroom. This is why it's vital to seek professional medical advice when making life-altering decisions that relate to your circadian rhythm.

A doctor's consultation, however, isn't always necessary. There are ways to get started that are safe for anyone to try.

Disclaimer: Some studies suggest that exposing bipolar patients to natural light in the morning may worsen their condition, as opposed to being exposed at midday, which seems to work well in resetting their clocks.

Before trying anything else, the best first step for any chronotype is to reset their circadian rhythm.

The reason why you need to do this is that most people's rhythms are out of alignment. They operate according to the hours dictated by their jobs or children's schedules etc. Meaning that if you have a job, it's probably best if you do this on a holiday.

Anyone (see disclaimer above) can do this safely, and the most effective reset method is through exposure to natural light. According to Dr Andrew Huberman, this is best done by stepping outside for at least 10 to 15 minutes each day in the morning within an hour of waking, preferably not wearing sunglasses – please do not look directly at the sun as this will damage your eyes, standing under a tree is sufficient – then repeating the same at dusk. Repeat this process for as many days as possible.

When outside, the ganglion cells in your eyes will interpret the type (tone, strength and colour) of light and inform your master clock what time of day it is. This will not work through the window, as light exposure through a window is 50 times less effective than outside. Also, most windows have filters that stop the ganglion cells from reading the light properly.

What's interesting is that being outside during sunset helps to protect your rhythm from synthetic lights, including devices, that you might be exposed to that same evening and night – not to mention the added benefit of vitamin D by exposure of your skin to sunlight.

In addition, limit your eating window to, preferably, between 8 to 10 hours (12 hours maximum), aligning it with the time you are most physically active. This includes not eating anything for at least an hour after waking up and having the last bite of food (that includes wine or caloric beverages) at least 3 to 4 hours before bedtime – although 5 to 6 hours is ideal, particularly after a heavy meal because it can take up to 6 hours for you to digest it. Also, research shows that eating a late meal, messes with the release of melatonin and other processes that are required to allow you to drift off to sleep; this further contributes to circadian rhythm misalignment.

Finally, try to avoid napping while attempting to reset your rhythm, unless absolutely necessary. Even then, try to limit the nap to a maximum of 30 minutes and not too late in the day. If you're not used to waking up early, you can experiment by progressively waking up slightly earlier (15 to 30 minutes each day) for a few weeks and see how that sits with your system; test how you feel cognitively and mentally, then adjust your hours accordingly. Who knows, maybe you're not a night owl after all.

The above steps will allow you to naturally reset and align with your genetic cycle and, hopefully, expose your true chronotype. However, if you're still unsure which category you belong to, there are other ways of identifying your chronotype. For example, get yourself tested at a reputable sleep clinic or a lab. Today, they can be found all over the globe and use psycho-physiological measures to identify your chronotype. These measures include circadian markers consisting of salivary and plasma melatonin and cortisol; electroencephalograph; cardio-metabolic indicators such as blood glucose and insulin levels; neuroendocrine secretion; and performance measures including cognitive and behavioural tests.

But if all of the above sounds like too much work and you want a quick and simple test that can easily narrow in on your genetic rhythm, you can fill out a *Composite Scale of Morningness* questionnaire. It was originally developed to identify evening types among university students. It's a quick form that can help anyone identify their chronotype. The form can be found online by googling its name: *composite scale of morningness.* Make sure to use double apostrophes at the start and at the end of the phrase to make your Google search easier.

Remember that the process of figuring out your chronotype may take some time. I've been living my (2:00 am to 9:30 am) routine for quite some time now, but it took almost 18 months of finetuning and listening to my body to get it right. Hopefully, you can learn from my mistakes and speed up this process.

When I first started my experiment, my bedtime quickly changed from 2 am to 3 am, then 4 am. This went on for months, and even though I was now getting around 6 hours of sleep a night – because I would naturally wake up around 9:30-10:00 am – which was an improvement from my 4 to 5 hour nights when I was working; however, I still wasn't feeling my best as 6 hours is about 2 hours short of what's recommended by sleep experts.

It wasn't until my husband and I went to visit our son in Melbourne that I accidentally, properly reset my body clock. You see, the guest room in his house had no curtains or blinds on the windows, so we slept fully exposed to the morning sun. It only took a few days; each day, I went to sleep earlier and earlier, finally settling back at around 2 am. The more significant change was that I was finally able to get over 7 hours of sleep each night. Still naturally waking up around 9:30 am.

I realised that it was the sun-blocking roller shutters fitted on the exterior of our bedroom windows back at home – which we closed shut every night – that initially slowly threw my body clock off: from 2 am bedtime to 4 am. Since that trip, we always leave about 50% of the roller shutters slightly open to let in the morning light. This small and almost insignificant change has allowed me to maintain my 2:00 am bedtime and 7 ½ hours sleeping schedule consistently (except pre-period – for more information, see chapter 3: female-specific issues).

The most important thing is that, once you find your routine, it's imperative that you stick to it. By that, I mean eat, exercise, work and go to sleep at the same time each day, and don't vary your hours on the weekend. In addition, try to get around 8 hours of sleep each night.

It's in your best interest to stick to a routine, but continue to listen to your body and, if necessary, make adjustments to your routine, but not too often. Remember that your body is continually evolving and changing. According to several studies, most night-owls' clocks advance as they age; meaning that you might start waking up slightly earlier with each year, starting as early as your mid-40s or early 50s.

How are night owls different?

One of the main differences between a morning person and a night owl – at a biological level – is their genes. For example, night owls have a shorter allele on the PER3 circadian clock gene. This gene is one of the primary components of the circadian clock system affecting rhythms of locomotor activity, metabolism and behaviour.

Another difference is the timing of the production and release of melatonin. Melatonin is a hormone produced by the pineal gland, typically released about 1 to 1.5 hours before you are due to fall asleep – i.e., when your master clock thinks is the optimal time for you to drift off to sleep. For owls, this hormone is released later on at night. This can vary from two to four hours later than the norm.

There's still a lot of mystery surrounding the exact role of melatonin; what we do know is that its release signals the arrival of night-time. Contrary to popular belief, melatonin does not make us sleep nor does it help us stay asleep. Although, there's strong evidence that shows when people ingest melatonin (in a form of a tablet or other), it helps them fall asleep faster.

Because melatonin is released later for night owls, it may be one of the reasons why, even when you try to go to sleep early, you can't fall asleep. It's because you don't have enough melatonin (at that time) to signal your brain that it's night-time. This is often the reason why night owls think they have insomnia.

The timing of your body's temperature is another major marker that seperates night owls from the rest. Because even though everyone's body temperature declines when it's time to go to sleep and rises when it's time to wake up, once again, this occurs a couple of hours later for night owls than for the rest of the population.

And finally, the timing of the rise of cortisol is another indicator that helps sleep clinicians establish your chronotype. This is because your body increases cortisol in order to wake you up naturally at the onset of your active phase.

It's important to note that no two chronological clocks are the same, and when I refer to night owls, I am speaking about a wide spectrum of people; some of them go to bed at midnight, some at 2 am, others at 4 am.

In the end, what all owls have in common is that they go to sleep later – or at least have a natural inclination to do so – than the rest of the population.

There are, of course, advantages to being a night owl. Let's start by debunking my least-favourite myth:

'The early bird catches the worm.'

Benjamin Franklin is famous for saying, 'Early to bed and early to rise makes a man wealthy, healthy and wise.' Some people thought it would be a good idea to test this hypothesis. So, Southampton University researchers Catharine Gale and Christopher Martyn followed a group of 356 morning larks and 318 night owls over a 20-year period and found that, while health seemed to be comparable across both groups, overall, the night owls were wealthier – i.e. had larger incomes – than the morning larks.

Also, some studies show that night owls have better emotional regulation, due to how their brains are wired – this is discussed later. However, other studies show the reverse is true. Although when reading the studies with adverse findings, it quickly becomes apparent that the tested night owls were studied under socially acceptable timeframes – meaning that they were in circadian misalignment – which might explain some of the negative conclusions.

Many studies also show that night owls score higher than morning people on general intelligence and creativity; however, morning larks get better grades at school.

In addition, night owls tend to have slightly less white matter (white matter helps neurons communicate); this means fewer pathways through which serotonin or dopamine – the feel-good hormones – can travel. This may explain why some studies find night owls are better at regulating emotions and have fewer addictive tendencies. But what they lack in white matter, they make up in cortisol – the stress hormone – which contributes to their get-things-done attitude and provides sustained energy that morning larks often have in low-supply, particularly towards the end of the day. However, the surplus of cortisol can sometimes lead to risk-taking. Meaning that night owls are more likely to take advantage of opportunities as they present themselves, resulting in greater financial gain or loss.

I would be doing you a disservice if I didn't mention the studies that claim the evening chronotype is associated with greater alcohol consumption, binge drinking and greater levels of alcohol dependence. Once again, there's plenty of evidence that these studies were carried out while the participants were in circadian misalignment, which, once again, explains the adverse findings.

***

In general terms, there are a number of physical and psychological characteristics that separate night owls from everyone else. One of the key differences is the timing of peak performance.

According to Dr Elise Facer-Childs, night owls peak on average 12 hours after waking – in both cognitive and physical tasks, as opposed to morning larks, who peak at cognitive tasks immediately after waking, and around seven hours after waking, at physical tasks. After which, their energy levels start to deteriorate rapidly as the evening approaches.

Once again, it is important to note that the night owls who participated in the above study were tested as early as 8 am during the study. In my opinion, is too early for most night owls, considering that the average night owl goes to sleep between 1 to 2 am, waking them up after only 6 to 7 hours of sleep could have potentially skewed the results.

Other studies show that both chronotypes perform equally well in reflection-time tests one hour after waking, but after ten hours of being awake, the night owl's energy is still high (and increasing), while the early lark's energy levels are on a downhill trajectory. So, even though morning types wake up full of energy, they cannot sustain that energy as long as the night owl, throughout the day.

Night owls at different stages of life

From infancy to about the age of 10, we all are skewered towards a morning rhythm. Then – most studies agree on this – all children progressively turn into night owls through adolescence, peaking in young adulthood – around the age of 16 to 18. However, our true genetic chronotype is usually revealed around the age of 20, that's when most people settle into the genetically driven rhythm that will stay with them for most of their adulthood.

Even though all teenagers are night owls, after the age of 18, the genetic morning types start to wake up earlier and earlier. The same goes for the intermediates although, they don't wake up as early as the larks; however, the night owls stay as they are. Although, as mentioned earlier, a good percentage of night owls slowly regresses back into an earlier rhythm as they age, turning into intermediates and, in some cases, into morning larks.

Ironically, the average time of death for morning people is around 11 am, while night owls' average time to say their final goodbye is around 6 pm.

Can night owls become early larks?

The next time somebody gives you the typical and not-so-helpful advice to 'Just try and go to sleep earlier', take them to a different time zone – one that's preferably 10 hours backwards or forwards – and say the same thing to them when they are lying awake at 3 am in the morning: 'Just try and go to sleep' and 'Why are you not trying?'. Maybe then, they'll understand what normal life for a night owl looks like, living in the early-riser society.

Please keep in mind that most people who are urging you to get up at 5 am because of how "good it is for you", are most likely doing it naturally. They usually make you feel guilty or try to prove their case for an early morning routine by claiming they also don't feel like getting up so early, but the truth is that they are naturally up at that time anyway, and what they mean by 'not feeling like getting up' is staying in bed to, for example, play on their phones or 'what have you'…

Dozens upon dozens of studies have proven that, given the chance to sleep *ad libitum* (as long as desired) and in alignment with their natural rhythm, most people wake up after about 8 hours, rested and ready to face the day, without a need for an alarm clock. So, don't buy into the stories about discipline. The fact is that most people who consistently wake up really early do it by choice and are natural early risers; their brain is a happy little birdy that is genetically wired to start the day at the crack of dawn.

> **Note**: if you have decided to take on the reset challenge and find that you're sleeping longer than 8 hours, this may be caused by one of 2 things. First, it's most likely that you have built up a sleep deficit and your body is trying to sleep off all those missed hours. Second, you just might happen to be one of those peo-

ple who naturally need an hour or two more than the norm. If it's the first one, the extra hours will persist for only a few days and soon you'll most likely fall into an 7 to 8 hour sleep pattern. If you happen to fall into the second catergory, try to embrace the extra hours, which may help to increase your creativity and improve your problem solving skills.

A word to the sceptic

Of course, not all morning people are like that. That's why I talked about the spectrum earlier, in that everybody's clock is a little different. But if you're already wired to get up at, say, 6 or 7 am, then 5 am is not such a huge stretch, and even though it might be a little uncomfortable for you, you can still function relatively well, having only shaved an hour or two from your sleep.

However, for a night owl, like me, who normally wakes up around 9:30 am, waking up at 5 am is the equivalent of waking a morning person just after midnight and asking them to get used to it: to repeat it day-in-day-out. Give them a shot of coffee and say, 'This should do. Now go exercise, have some brekky and at 1 am, go to work and be happy and alert for the next 8 hours. Then, come home, make dinner, do the dishes, help the kids with homework...' – I'm hoping you get the picture. If that happened, we would have a society of zombies unable to utter logical words to one another; we would turn into a society of imbeciles, and our society would collapse as we know it.

Please understand that when a night owl doesn't want to wake up in the morning, it isn't because we dislike it (although we do: we loathe it) or because we lack discipline: it's because we are literally unable to function.

When we wake up that early, what you see is just a show, a shell walking around with a pretend smile and an automated 'Hello, how are you?'. Let me assure you, the moment you turn around, we crawl into a corner in the closest office cubicle and rock ourselves back and forth while crying uncontrollably, dreading tomorrow because we know that we have to do it all over again.

Chapter Four

Body

Your master clock predicts the future

Your body does not like to deal with things ad-hoc. It is always prepared, even for the unexpected. For example, when you cut yourself, your system has pre-designed processes in place to stop the bleeding, to protect you against infection and optimise the healing process. Your immune system carries a list of every illness or germ it has ever encountered, ready to attack any invaders on and off that list.

In essence, your body is nothing more than a walking, talking, predicting machine. And the main function of the master clock is to assist the body in making those predictions, including when you should eat, sleep, go to work, exercise, be creative or solve problems.

The clock's job is to anticipate, design and initiate processes to help your system cope with the range of activities it has predicted that you'll face at different times of the day. Those essential processes are a series of highly orchestrated events that deal with metabolism, hormones, temperature, mood etc. and operate in sequence within the 24-hour cycle.

For example, as your time to wake up approaches, your clock prepares your body for the active phase by raising cortisol and your body temperature while depleting the rest of the adenosine (sleep pressure) that's flowing through your system.

And while the stomach lining is regenerated each night – which prevents the digestive juices and enzymes from eating through the stomach walls – as soon as you wake up, the clock is anticipating when you're going to start eating so it can initiate the processes, such as increasing ghrelin (the hunger hormone) and saliva production, and other systems that allow your digestive system to convert food into energy and nutrients for your body.

Your body is continuously predicting your energy demand at any given time during the active phase and releases the appropriate amount of glucose (energy) it thinks you will need to accomplish your daily tasks.

This means that when you're awake and consuming food while in misalignment with your body clock – i.e., while your circadian rhythm is in a rest phase – you not only disrupt the stomach lining restoration process, you also miss out on the intake of nutrients, which in that state greatly reduced or close to non-existent, according to Hans Reinke PhD, a researcher at the University of Duesseldorf in Germany.

The inability to absorb nutrients reduces the amount of energy you're able to produce. In addition, inadequate absorption of nutrients inhibits oxygen consumption, which would otherwise generate carbon dioxide – required for proper metabolic regulation.

This explains why night owls feel so lethargic when they wake up early, even when they have a nutritious breakfast. It's because their body is in sleep mode and isn't ready to initiate the required processes for you to take advantage of the nutrients and energy you had just consumed.

Of course, the reduction in energy during the rest phase has its purpose. The 'saving' of energy during the allocated sleep cycle allows the body to 'spend' it on a myriad of protective, regenerative, adaptive and anabolic processes – such as immune functions, synaptic plasticity and glycogen storage.

What's more, rest-phase processes allow your brain to consolidate your memories and emotions – what's going on behind the scenes is a huge clean-up and dumping of irrelevant information, immortalising new relevant information and updating old memory files, in case any new information is relevant to your understanding of what happened, or what you've experienced or learned, in the past.

In fact, your entire system, that is, every cell in your body, goes through a reset and rejuvenation process during your sleep cycle.

Studies show that for every hour your body is regularly out of sync with your circadian rhythm, you increase the risk of obesity between 30% to 50%, which in turn increases the risk of other diseases such as diabetes, high blood pressure, cardiovascular disease and sleep apnoea. You're also 30% more likely to develop various forms of cancer, particularly hormonal cancers, in addition to severely disabling your immune system. In fact, a 2018 study shows a much higher occurrence of colorectal cancer in nurses working night shift, caused by circadian rhythm misalignment, since most people are day-dwellers, which is why the International Agency for Research on Cancer has classified night-shift work as category 2A: probable carcinogen.

Not getting enough sleep causes you to consume more food because the hormone responsible for making you feel satiated, leptin, is diminished, while the hormone responsible for making you feel hungry, ghrelin, is amplified. In fact, according to world-leading chronobiology scientist Professor Russell Foster of Oxford University, individuals who live in constant misalignment with their body clock or who regularly don't get enough sleep have higher levels of ghrelin (up to 24%), and lower levels of leptin (as much as 18%), which contributes to weight gain and increases their probability of developing metabolic diseases.

Getting enough sleep that is synchronised with your rhythm also supports a healthy microbiome, which allows your body to regulate your appetite and helps you to make better food choices.

Studies in recent years show that body clock misalignment changes the microbiome, making it a more hostile environment for beneficial gut bacteria while increasing the number of unhealthy gut bacteria. This has a direct impact on metabolism and immune response; it can even accelerate the aging process.

In addition, night owls who live in misalignment with their chronotype consistently show higher C-reactive protein, a marker for higher inflammation in the body. Inflammation is your body's natural way of protecting you, helping you heal from an infection, injury or disease. However, when it lasts too long, it becomes chronic and starts to damage healthy tissues. Chronic inflammation is associated with a plethora of health problems, including heart disease, diabetes, cancer, arthritis and bowel diseases, like Crohn's disease and ulcerative colitis.

The anatomy of sleep

Most studies report that, given the opportunity, an average healthy adult will sleep between 7 to 8 hours, if not disturbed. However, a 4-year (2003–07) US study of over 56,000 individuals aged between 18 and 64 found that women, on average, get slightly more sleep than men: around 15 minutes.

And while some people think that the brain goes into a rest mode at night, they might be surprised to find out that even though you're asleep, your brain is a hub of activity. Guy Leschziner, a professor of Neurology and Sleep Medicine at King's College in London, says that some areas of the brain become even more active at night than they are during the day.

A normal 8-hour sleep progresses in 70 to 90-minute cycles. Each cycle consists of two types of sleep: non-rapid eye movement (NREM) and rapid eye movement (REM). Both NREM and REM, are essential.

NREM sleep, otherwise known as slow-wave sleep, helps with learning and allows your brain to remove unnecessary neuro connections and clear your 'cache' by 'downloading' your memory from a temporary storage space (in the hippocampus) to a permanent, long-term memory storage (temporal neocortex), the 'hard drive' of your brain.

There is something beautiful about what happens during NREM sleep; it can be compared to the brain 'watching' a movie of your most recent memories and deleting what it deems unimportant or trivial, such as the exact colour of the flowers you passed on your way to work. It also matches and updates any past memories that are relevant to your recent experiences, expanding your understanding of the world.

REM sleep is also amazing as this is when the important neuro connections are strengthened. This phase of the sleep cycle is all about creativity and problem-solving, but it also helps you to manage your emotions. The phrase 'I'll sleep on it' when faced with making a difficult decision is there for a reason, but you need plenty of REM sleep to help you make the best decision.

NREM (slow wave) sleep always proceeds REM sleep, but they are not spread equally within the 90-minute cycle. NREM dominates the sleeping cycles for the first few hours, with only a small proportion of each cycle allocated to REM sleep. However, in the last 2 to 3 hours of sleep – within an 8-hour sleep timeframe – it is REM that dominates the 70 to 90-minute sleep cycle.

This means that consistently losing 2 hours of sleep, as is the case for most night owls, isn't just a simple case of math: 25% loss of sleep. What actually happens is they lose about 80% of REM sleep – the very sleep that is critical for creativity, emotional well-being and your ability to solve problems a.k.a. 'sleeping on it'.

Insomnia and early death

Studies show that consistently going against your natural circadian rhythm will shorten your life – in some cases, considerably. Walker also says that consistently under-sleeping may, in rare cases, cause *progressive insomnia*, which usually manifests itself midlife. This type of insomnia is incurable and culminates in the patient's inability to sleep altogether, which ends in early death. While the initial phase of this ailment can take many years, the final process takes between 12 to 18 months, severely shortening the life of its victims.

Many night owls think that they have insomnia because there are unable to fall asleep when they go to bed at an 'appropriate time', but this is common, so don't be alarmed if this happens to you. Instead, try going to bed a little later each day and see how fast you're able to fall asleep then. If you're still lying awake, try a little later time the next day. If you keep on experimenting, you'll finally find your sweet spot, and if your lifestyle permits, you will also be able to enjoy at least 7 to 8 hours of sleep, depending on your age and your state of health.

Female-specific issues

To start, a woman's biological rhythm becomes fixed around 19.5 years of age. It is about this time that most of your peers, who, as teenagers, could party all night long, start going to sleep earlier, suddenly making you the only one holding up your hand for a late-night movie marathon.

Women generally enjoy better sleep quality than men. For example, on average, they're able to fall asleep faster and sleep for longer; their sleep is also deeper. However, women experience slightly more sleep disorders, such as insomnia or restless leg syndrome. They also have higher instances of sleep disturbances caused by puberty, periods, pregnancy, and menopause.

For many women, their menstrual cycle is one of the biggest sleep disruptors, which can completely mess up their rhythm just before the onset of the period. It may be several days before they bounce back into their natural circadian rhythm. If you're a woman, it's important to take this into consideration when conducting your chronotype evaluation or reset. You don't want to observe your pre-period late nights and accidentally misidentify yourself as a night owl when you normally fall asleep at a socially acceptable hour on other days of the month.

***

Several studies have shown that sleeping deficit causes polycystic ovaries. This leads to an overproduction of testosterone, which, apart from messing with your menstrual cycle, contributes to the development of masculine characteristics, such as excess body hair.

Also, several studies show a much higher occurrence of breast cancer in rotating shift-working nurses.

What's more, poor sleep quality or rhythm misalignment may reduce fertility by altering the levels of reproductive hormones. This is especially prevalent in female shift workers, who have a much higher percentage of infertility when compared to their diurnal counterparts. Studies also show that circadian misalignment can contribute to higher incidences of recurrent miscarriages.

Your circadian rhythm also plays an important role in child-rearing; it can even affect the timing of labour onset. As it turns out, your master clock will take into consideration the best time that you'll be able to sustain the energy required to go through labour and give birth. Interestingly, all of my labours (I have four children) started either late afternoon or evening, which is perfect timing considering that all my labours lasted between 6 to 12 hours.

Male-specific issues

As mentioned earlier, men get an average of 15 minutes less sleep per day than women. However, studies show that this is not biologically driven. It turns out that men get less sleep because they're more likely to choose entertainment, like watching TV, over going to sleep early. It may not seem like much, but if this is the only habit you could improve, you'd be on your way to *significantly* improving your mood and health – particularly when that extra sleep is aligned with your chronotype.

Of course, there are other benefits of well-aligned 8-hour sleep, such as a healthy libido and well-adjusted testosterone levels.

According to a 2022 study (and others), Chronological misalignment can cause a lot of trouble in bed. This ranges from erectile dysfunction to reduced penis girth and hardness. It also affects your libido.

For those who are planning a family, poor sleep routine can reduce sperm count and overall production and cause certain cancers, including prostate cancer. In some cases, ongoing sleep deprivation causes infertility.

Other sleeping-related statistics that are different for men is that they are much more likely to be affected by the rapid eye movement sleep behaviour disorder and the Kleine-Levin syndrome.

And finally, a man's biological rhythm settles around the age of 21, a little later than it does for a woman (around 19.5 years of age).

Chapter Five

Mind

Living in an early-riser society

When a night owl tries to fit in the world of the early riser, they have to battle both their *physiology* and *psychology*.

On the physical side, the misalignment is causing chronic sleep deprivation, which, on any given day feels like you have the clarity of a zombie, and your body is continually fighting a strong dose of horse tranquiliser. In addition to the physical strain, your psychology is also suffering, which can lead to long-term mental health issues. These issues are mainly caused by the adverse biochemical factors, which play a major role affecting your neuro-processing.

This is on top of an ongoing monologue with which night owls often crucify themselves; this includes phrases such as 'I'm lazy', 'I'm irresponsible', 'I'm useless' and 'what in the world is wrong with me?!'

According to Sean Drummond, a clinical neuroscientist and professor at Monash University, your ability to process emotions and your reaction to things going on around you are altered when you're running on a sleep deficit.

For the most part, you're more irrational and react quicker (and more strongly) than if you had a good night's sleep. Even an hour less sleep per day, over three or more days, will result in increased bad decision-making, reduced impulse control and inability to focus.

In addition, Prof Russell Foster of Oxford University says circadian misalignment causes you to lose empathy because it prevents you from picking up on subtle social cues communicated through facial expressions or body language – a skill that's essential to developing and maintaining healthy relationships with others.

It will also cause mood swings and irritability. And if the above isn't enough, Foster adds that circadian rhythm disruption makes you much more likely to engage in risky behaviour and to make impulsive, unreflective decisions.

Many studies show that for every 2 hours your body is regularly out of sync with your circadian rhythm, you more than double the risk of severe depression. One of the causes might be that, according to Prof Foster, when misalignment (or sleep loss) occurs, we tend to forget positive experiences and interpret our reality through our negative memories.

This was recently confirmed by a 2021 UK study of over 85,000 people. It found that when night owls work during hours misaligned with their natural rhythm, they are significantly more likely to develop depression, anxiety and, in some cases, other mental health issues such as schizophrenia, Alzheimer's and bipolar disease.

In the end, aligning your active-rest periods with your master clock is not just about avoiding mental health issues; it's the fact that a person who is in sync with their circadian rhythm has an overall better sense of well-being, meaning they're a lot healthier and happier.

Neurological deterioration

World-leading sleep expert Matthew Walker says that operating outside of one's chronocycle causes neural degeneration. Typically, neural degeneration is intrinsically connected with age-related decline, which translates to chronic diseases and cognitive deterioration, including dementia. However, this process is immensely accelerated for shift workers that's because they regularly operate out of sync with their circadian rhythm and are often chronically sleep-deprived.

Neuroscientists studying the brains of shift workers say that, over a 10-year span, a shift worker's neural degeneration is 6.5 years more advanced than that of a non-shift worker. In more simple terms, for every 10 years, a shift worker ages 16.5 years.

***

One of the processes that occurs *only* while we sleep is best described as a 'brain shower'. This 'shower' occurs when the cerebrospinal fluid enters the brain during NREM (deep) sleep.

You see, the brain doesn't have a lymphatic system, which is present everywhere else in your body and serves to remove toxins and other impurities from your system. So, the scientist think that this nightly 'shower' is an alternative way to clear the brain of toxins and other waste. This is particularly important in the case of preventing dementia since its most common cause is plaque build-up in the brain. Now, there is still a lot that the scientists don't know about the purpose of this nightly brain shower, but what they do know is that when you cut back on your sleep, you reduce your brain's ability to rid itself from this build-up and increase your chances of cognitive decline.

Cognitive impairment

So much of our daily life – particularly working life – is spent creating, remembering, problem-solving and making decisions, all of which require a well-functioning cognitive capacity. Yet, according to Sabina Brennan, a neuroscientist and author of *Beating brain fog*, about 600 million people around the globe regularly suffer from loss of mental clarity – science calls it 'cognitive dysfunction'.

This is, of course, of great importance to us on an individual level, but also on a collective level. Some of the worse disasters in human history are attributed to 'morning people' functioning in misalignment with their biological clock by working the night shift. These disasters include the Chernobyl nuclear explosion, the space shuttle *Challenger* tragedy and the Alaskan oil spill.

Your brain is a dominant consumer of the overall energy produced by your body and uses about a quarter of the nutrients you intake. Brennan says that your body loves patterns and routine because it's trying to optimise – to save energy. This means that your brain isn't always 'on' – sometimes it's in 'sleep mode', even when you're awake. By tracking your daily routine, your master clock plans ahead when that brain energy is going to be required, and as long as it aligns with your circadian wake-time (active phase), it will make that energy available when you need it.

A 2018 study led by Sarah Chellappa PhD, a neuroscientist at the University of Cologne, shows that circadian misalignment doesn't just slow down our reaction time and impede our ability to focus and process information; it also prevents us from learning new things.

***

If you are enjoying this book so far, it would mean so much to me if you could write a quick review; this could help others decide whether this book is for them.

Chapter Six

Work

Career

Living in an early-riser society puts the night owl at a disadvantage, particularly from a social perspective, because they are in a constant state of what scientists call 'social jetlag'.

This is particularly evident in one's work life and begins even before you start a new job. That's because first impressions really count and when you get slotted-in for an early-morning interview, you are significantly reducing your chances of making that first impression the best it could be.

The next thing that suffers is your work relationships. That's because waking up early makes you extra groggy and often puts you in a foul mood – not the best recipe for building lasting relationships, this includes both your colleagues and customers.

In a perfect world and all things being equal, a night owl should be able to have their cake and eat it too; meaning, you should have the ability to sleep according to your biological rhythm while being able to pursue the career of your dreams. This is, obviously, not always possible in today's society, so how can you navigate this problem?

First of all, you have to ask yourself a number of questions that take into account your **worldview**, your **situation** and your **values**.

Worldview

Being human, you already have a formed worldview about your work life. Most people that I speak to about this, think that a night owl just has to suck it up and sacrifice their sleep and health for work. They say it's 'being realistic'. As you know, until recently, I shared that worldview. However, the great thing about a worldview is that you can change it. This means that you have a few options.

First, you could either choose a path of self-employment, like I have, giving you flexibility over your working hours or choose a career path that allows you to work in alignment with your rhythm. You might be surprised how many options are available to you that go well beyond the obvious, such as a security guard, concierge or nurse. I recently saw a job post for a white-collar position for an Evening/Night Shift Administrator in a nursing home.

Second, if the career of your dreams is typically a morning person's job, you might think that you're out of options. But the truth is that increasingly more and more employers are now offering flexible working hours and work-from-home options for their workforce.

Third, if you're already in a job you like, you can talk to your current employer to see if they would be willing to negotiate your hours or allow you to work from home, which would eliminate the morning commute and the time required to get yourself looking presentable, giving you extra time for sleep.

Finally, if you're reading this and you happen to be a business owner or someone in charge of HR decisions concerning working hours, please consider amending your policies and employment contracts to accommodate your employees' chronotypes. And not just for the night owls. Today's standard working hours fall outside of the norm even for the intermediates, with many jobs starting as early as 7 am. Much too early for about 70% of the population (comprising night owls 20% and intermediates 50%), considering that a 7 am start often equals a 5 am wake-up routine; to allow sufficient time to shower, dress, eat and travel to work.

Situation

Having said all of the above, your worldview can be greatly impacted by your current situation – e.g., financial, family or even your age.

For example, the younger you are, the more options you have because you may have fewer commitments, such as a family or a mortgage. You're also still in the early stages of your career, meaning that you haven't yet invested years into a certain field, making it easier for you to make a switch.

The older you get, the more likely it is that you have spent years cultivating a career and reputation in a niche area. You are also more likely to be further along on the corporate ladder, making it harder for you to switch, especially if you're the only breadwinner and have a family to support.

Values

What is important to you? Do you care about your looks or your health? Or how long you are going to live? Being a night owl, you have to ask yourself some questions about what you are willing to sacrifice now to ensure a better future. Do you mind having to rely on medication or the help of your loved ones to take care of you because of illness (long-term)?

I know that the statistics provided by the hundreds of studies are not very emotional; they are just numbers on a page, but that's until you become that number and think, why didn't I do anything when I had the chance?

How hard are you prepared to fight for your future? Or maybe I should put it this way: it might seem like a huge change right now, but in the end, once you do what's required to ensure your chronotype is aligned with your work and lifestyle, when you look back, it might not seem like a huge sacrifice. Especially, when you realise how great you feel: living with elevated energy, increased cognitive clarity and a renewed zest for life. This is what happened to me, and it feels great!

Some people, however, choose to ignore their biological rhythm and power through. And even though I read about these people in studies and research papers, nothing brings it home the same way as seeing the effects of living in misalignment played out on someone I know. My friend, with whom I used to be very close for many years, has worked her entire life as a nurse. She is a natural morning lark, yet her job often required her to work the night shift. As a single mum, she felt that she was out of options and pushed through. Long story short, I met up with her recently after about a 10-year gap of not seeing each other. I was in utter horror at what I saw. The thing is that even though I read all those studies talking about accelerated aging, and I was able to process the statistics, seeing it with my own eyes gave me a completely different perspective. At 56 and only 8 years older than me, she looked like a 70-year-old grandmother. In fact, many 70-year-olds look better. At that moment, I was so grateful that I decided to bite the bullet and leave my successful construction career behind.

The accelerated aging might not mean much to men, but to us, girls, this particularly hits home because our looks are important to us, and we work hard to maintain our youthful appearance for as long as possible.

***

I understand that switching careers, or in some cases going from an employee to self-employment, might seem scary: it is, after all, a question of financial security and stability, and for some, even reputation. However, you don't have to go all in; you can gradually transition to another way of life. Maybe set aside a time, a few times a week to work on a side hustle that might eventually turn into a source of full-time income.

Also, before you make any changes, it's a good idea to figure out your true chronotype. I suggest taking time out (leave from work) or using a holiday to experiment going to bed in alignment with your natural rhythm. Try waking up at different hours of the morning and remember to expose yourself to natural sunlight within the first half hour of waking. And give the experiment some time to settle because, remember, your entire system is out of whack, and it will take time (up to 2 weeks) to adjust and align your clock.

For me, I eventually settled on going to bed between 1:00 and 2:00 am, but this doesn't mean that I don't have bad nights anymore; I do. Sometimes I can't fall asleep until 5 or 6 am. Some of this is because I am a woman, and my menstrual cycle impacts my sleeping pattern (see section on female-specific issues). Sometimes, it's simply because I just have too many ideas flying around in my brain, and I can't stop playing with them. Regardless of the reason, I always try to get myself back on track as soon as I can by going to bed at the same time and following a strict morning routine, because I know it's the optimum rhythm for my health, productivity and emotional stability.

Physical work

Your body clock affects how well you perform at both mental and physical tasks at different times of the day. A new study at Monash University headed by Dr Facer-Child reveals that night owls have an 8.4% slower reaction time in the morning than their early-chronotype colleagues.

Another study led by Monash University's Associate Professor Clare Anderson shows that fatigue (induced by insufficient sleep) causes 20% of car accidents and 11% of fatalities on Victorian roads (Australia). This statistic is echoed by other studies around the world.

These figures have great implications for accidents at work, particularly for those operating heavy machinery or jobs requiring high levels of cognitive and physical precision, e.g., surgeons. This is why the best work for night owls, who prefer physical work, is something that involves a later start – preferably an afternoon shift – because it's not just your own safety at risk, but the safety of others.

Cognitive work

Being a white-collar employee gives you much more flexibility in today's workplace, particularly in light of Covid lockdowns, which made remote work commonplace and much more accepted by employers.

If your current employer isn't able to accommodate your night-owl tendencies, you might want to look for remote work with employers who are happy for you to work outside of normal office hours, or employers based in time zones that align with your later-in-the-day routine.

However, Andrea Valeria, a career specialist for remote workers, says that when you're job-hunting, transparency is king and that it's best to be upfront about your 'operating' hours.

If you absolutely cannot get out of a standard 9–5, Dr Carmel Harrington, author of *The Sleep Diet*, suggests that night owls should do the most creative and taxing work after midday. Leaving the morning for more automated tasks, such as email checking. And from mid-morning, progressively transitioning to more cognitively demanding tasks, such as making phone calls, placing orders, updating databases etc.

You can also communicate your preferences to people responsible for setting meeting times by asking that, if possible, they aren't held first thing in the morning. However, be mindful that this may impact how you are perceived by those working above you. Studies have found that implicit and explicit bias against night owls from management in the workplace can diminish a night owl's ability to advance their career because they are often seen as lazy and irresponsible, simply by requesting for a task or a meeting to be delayed based on their chronotype-specific needs. This obviously does not apply to all people, so depending on the person you're dealing with as well as your situation and career aspirations, you might want to refrain from any comments about your scheduling preferences, which is obviously not the narrative in this book, but that may be your reality.

In the end, before you decide how to schedule your workday, just remember that we are all different, so even when you observe two night owls of the same gender and same age who share identical bedtime schedules, it's likely that their energy and cognitive peaks and lows will happen at slightly different at times during the day. You are unique, and what you consider a light task, another night owl might deem demanding at an identical time of the day. For example, I've met night owls that can easily hold a conversation as soon as they open their eyes in the morning, where I'm barely able to utter a single word; yet I'm quite happy to perform semi-demanding physical tasks like making my bed, doing some light gardening or going for a short walk.

Athletes

Dr Elise Facer-Childs, founder of *Peak Sleep to Elite* which provides consulting services to top sports bodies around the world, says that **sleep is the most underutilised performance enhancer!**

Her studies show that understanding your chronotype and knowing when you're more likely to peak could literally mean the difference between a gold medal and coming in last. Since night owls are more likely to peak later on in the day, it might pay – if possible – to organise your athletic endeavours during more favourable hours.

Also, in her recent study, she says that there is a direct link between poor sleep and adverse mental health outcomes. The problem is that athletes, who are under constant pressure to perform at the highest level, often hide or underreport their mental health struggles. She suggests that sleep assessments should become an ongoing part of routine health and rehabilitation programs in sports.

In addition, two studies – one in 2017 and another in 2020 – showed the impact of the *skeletal muscle clock* on regulating **metabolic** and **hypoxic** stress during strenuous exercise.

> Metabolic and hypoxic stress: diminished blood flow causing insufficient amount of oxygen and glucose delivered to the tissues.

For example, the muscle glucose uptake during excercise can be up to 30 to 50 times higher than what's required during rest. When compromised, the skeletal muscle clock's capacity to regulate these processes is greatly reduced and, at times, impaired. In plain terms, a disrupted circadian rhythm will diminish your body's ability to deal with the physical demands of performing at your best.

Another study in 2022 by a team of researchers at Northwestern University in Chicago shows that disrupting the circadian rhythm adversely affects recovery after injury, including the speed and extent of recovery. This is huge for professional athletes as it affects how quickly they are able to start training again after an injury or how well that injury can heal and not cause issues in the future.

Entrepreneurs

One of the biggest perks of being self-employed is that you have the advantage of setting your own 'business hours'. In my business as a freelance writer, I'm always very upfront with my clients about my schedule. I manage their expectations even before they hire me. I do this by letting them know that they are unlikely to hear back right away if they send me an email in the morning, I also let them know that my phone is always switched off until about 10 am and when I say, 'I'll submit my work by the end of the day', what I mean is very late that night or early morning (1 or 2 am) the following day. This has helped me to avoid any schedule-related problems with my clients because they know exactly what to expect when choosing my services.

Another great tip, if your business is listed on Google Maps, is to adjust the trading hours to reflect your availability.

As a night owl, it is also best to set all your client meetings for the afternoon. This will allow you to be fully engaged and present for the client.

***

Congrats! You've made it to about the halfway mark – what do you think of this book so far? If you haven't already done it, I'd love it if you could write a quick review on your chosen platform or invite me for a podcast interview ;)

Chapter Seven

Parenting

Newborns and young children

Becoming a parent is a challenge for all parents in that most of them experience at some degree of sleep deficit. Before I had my first child, I remember someone telling me that I won't be able to get any sleep at night, to which I thought, 'No problem, I don't sleep at night anyway.' What they didn't mention is that I will not be able to get much sleep during the day either, which, in hindsight, should've been obvious to me.

While sleep deprivation caused by a newborn is temporary, lasting anywhere from a few weeks to about a year (some of us are luckier than others), the biggest test for night owls comes when their offspring enter the education system. Getting your children ready for school in the morning and dropping them off can be quite taxing for a night owl, and it lasts for years – right up until they get their own driver's licence and are finally able to get around independently.

There are several solutions to this challenge. The most obvious is to inquire about home-schooling solutions offered in your country; that's if your financial situation allows you to stay at home or if you're able to enter into a work-from-home arrangement with your employer. This way, you can start 'school' for your children a little later in the day.

If that's not an option, you can ask your partner or other non-night-owl family member to take over or help you in the morning in exchange for other duties you might be able to offer (later on in the day) to reduce their daily load.

Ultimately, if you have no support, doing anything that can allow you to sleep a little longer and decrease the time required to get your children ready in the morning will translate into significant cognitive, emotional and physical benefits for you for the remainder of the day. This includes doing as much as you can the night before. For example, making lunches and getting their (and your) clothes ready. You might even consider creating a checklist that you and your children, depending on their age, might check off to move things along more swiftly in the morning.

> Keep in mind that, if you are a night owl, one or more of your children is likely to inherit this gene set from you, although this will not become evident until young adulthood – from about 18 to 21 years of age.

However, I want to warn you against changing your children's routine to align with your own; for example, putting them to sleep slightly later, hoping they will wake up later and let you catch up on sleep. This is not a good idea as all preadolescent children have a disposition towards an earlier rhythm, and a delayed sleep schedule can be harmful not just in the present but can adversely impact their development. A New Zealand study of 341 preadolescent children found that circadian clock misalignment is strongly linked with excessive weight, particularly in girls.

Adolescents

In today's society, the notion of waking up sleepy and repeatedly hitting the snooze button is deemed 'normal'. This might be the reason why we are not alarmed when we hear statistics about the 80% of adolescents who wake up feeling this way. We think this is part of life, that it's 'supposed' to be this way.

This is such a common phenomenon that it's depicted in almost every movie about adolescents. You know the scene where the 'responsible' parent enters their teenager's room saying, 'Wake up honey, get ready for school,' to which the teenager inaudibly mumbles something and turns to the other side, trying to get at least a few more minutes of shut-eye. We don't do this to babies; why are we doing it to our teenagers?

We don't shake the baby when it's taking a nap by saying 'wake up, you lazy monkey, it's daytime, why are you asleep?!' No, this would be considered crazy or, possibly, even child abuse. Instead, we try to stay quiet and let the baby sleep because we understand how important sleep is to an infant's development process; not to mention that we don't want to put up with the drama of what would follow such a rude awakening.

The disadvantage that adolescents have is that, by now, they have developed some level of social skills and restraint (some more than others) and won't start screaming at the top of their lungs in protest. Most understand the importance of education and its role in their future, so they begrudgingly hold their tongue and force themselves out of bed.

***

From the age of about 10, the hormonal changes responsible for puberty cause a temporary change in children: they all gradually turn into varying degrees of night owls.

Study after study shows that **all** teenagers are night owls. This is confirmed by biological markers, such as body temperature, timing of melatonin release etc. It also means that no amount of parental threats will make them go to sleep earlier, no matter how hard they try. During this stage of their development, your child's (temporary) circadian rhythm will let them fall asleep, on average, no earlier than between midnight and 2 am.

It means that if you wake up your teenager at 6 am, they are only able to get around 4 to 6 hours of sleep. Experts call this sleep drunkenness. It impaires the student's ability to concentrate and absorb information, negatively impacting academic results. According to B-Society, ALL schools that have delayed starting times for teenagers and young adults have reported improved grades (especially for females).

Reduced sleep doesn't just reduce your adolescent's academic capabilities; it also diminishes their ability to responsibly drive a car. Monash University researchers in Australia found that drivers who had little sleep are 10 times as likely to be involved in a car accident.

According to Matthew Walker, allowing your child to go to sleep and wake up later – to align with this temporary rhythm change – will significantly reduce aggression and assist them with better decision-making, which is essential for teenagers, particularly in peer-pressure situations. It will also make your high-schooler more emotionally resilient and much nicer to live with.

Some believe that teenagers go to sleep later because the older the child gets, the less sleep they need, not taking into account the change in their circadian rhythm. Some of the world's most prominent sleep organisations, such as the National Sleep Foundation, recommend that 14 to 17-year-olds get at least 8 to 10 hours of sleep a night. This drops to about 8 to 9 hours at the age of 18. This is also when the circadian rhythm starts to recede the clock in about 80% of the youth but remains the same for the other 20%. This is basically the age when you find out whether you are a genetic night owl or a day-dweller.

So if your teenager consistently gets less than the prescribed amount of sleep, the missing hours – mostly composed of REM sleep, crucial in your child's brain development (of the frontal cortex) – are lost. And, as mentioned earlier, the frontal cortex is the brain's reasoning centre. It's where rational decision-making takes place. By letting your child miss out on those last 2 to 3 hours of sleep, you are actively taking away their ability to make sound, well-considered decisions, on an ongoing basis. Scientists have only been able to measure the effects of sleep deprivation in short-term studies – days or a few weeks. However, there are other studies that explore the long-term effects of adolescent sleep deprivation, which often translate into life-long consequences, most of which are associated with emotional instability (in some cases schizophrenia, discussed further on), or even criminal activity. But in most cases, continuous sleep deprivation of adolescents and young adults reduces their chances of eventually being able to live as a fully functioning adult member of society.

***

Coming back to the immediate effects of sleep deficit, the first thing that happens is that it negatively affects your child's mood, making them cranky and unsociable – not the best recipe for making or keeping friends. Even if they try to follow the best strategies from the author of *How to make friends and influence people*, their sleep drunkenness will impact their capacity to socialise and maintain relationships.

Lack of sleep hits teenagers three-fold: neurologically, physically and mentally. First, it impairs their attention and memory. Second, it increases the risk of obesity, weakens their immune system and reduces performance – for example, in school sports. And third, it affects their mood by increasing aggression and depressive tendencies, negatively impacting their social interactions.

Because this affects some adolescents more than others, the effects can range from mild to extreme; from lowered academic results to being expelled from school to using drugs and alcohol as a coping mechanism. In extreme cases, prolonged sleep deprivation results in suicidal behaviour and schizophrenia – particularly in young males.

In fact, many studies now show a direct link between the onset of schizophrenia – in young males around the age of 18 to 20 – and sleep deprivation.

***

Some schools around the world are already implementing measures to navigate this serious issue, by either delaying school starting times for adolescents or offering options for students to start at different times on different days. This issue has made its impact on government policy. For example, in the US, California was the first state to pass a law in 2019 to protect adolescent sleep health. Some countries list adolescent sleep deprivation as a significant risk in preventing and fighting diseases.

But the solutions come with obvious challenges, such as working parents' schedules, additional burdens on teachers etc. The real question is that even if the schools adjust their times accordingly, would the schedules of parents allow these students to sleep in? As we know, many working parents wake up their kids around 5 am, dropping them off at out-of-hours school care (OHSC) centres, to make it to work on time.

These are questions only the parents can answer. Every person's situation is different, but what I hope to achieve with this book is to give you, the parent, the ability to make an informed decision while weighing all the pros and cons that apply in your particular case.

When there are no other options but to get your adolescent out of bed in the early hours of the morning, there are a few tools at your disposal to manage the challenge. A 2020 study led by Svetlana Maskevich, a psychologist and PhD candidate at Monash University, shows promising results for better outcomes by planning around bedtimes.

The first of these options includes stress management. Stress has been found to be a big factor in your teenager's ability to get a good night's sleep, with what Maskevich calls 'pre-sleep arousal' – the main culprit for poor sleep. You can greatly reduce that stress by limiting the use of technological devices during evening-night hours. She found that the use of such devices at night may lead to the immature adjustment function of your child's master clocks.

Other options (which I've already listed in the section on *Newborns and young children*) include preparing as much as possible the night before. For example, laying out the clothes and having the school bag packed and ready for the next day; having an easily accessible simple morning checklist; preparing breakfast the night before, preferably one that can be consumed on the way to school. Each and every task that's necessary to get your child to school that can be prepared the night before, thus increasing their sleep time, makes a huge difference to their ability to be productive and effective that day.

Chapter Eight

Life

This section is dedicated to the 'day in the life' of a night owl. It talks about everyday things we all do, reinterpreted to suit the life of evening types.

I have tried to cover as many areas as possible, but if I have missed anything, just remember to plan your day according to your energy levels. For example, even though you might feel refreshed in the morning, be mindful that your cognitive ability and reasoning ability is still getting warmed up, so don't make important decisions first thing after getting out of bed. Also, because you're at a much higher risk of injury, refrain from heavy workouts early in the day; rather, spend this time on simple, light activities that can be performed on autopilot. Activities requiring the most energy are best carried out during your fully warmed up active phase: 2 to 3 hours after waking all the way to late evening. Creative tasks are best left for the end of the day when the owl's brain is most active.

Most importantly, remember that, unlike the left- and right-hand analogy, your chronotype isn't fixed for life, and many owls become increasingly larkish as they age. Make sure you monitor yourself as you age, particularly after your mid-40's, and make the necessary adjustments to your lifestyle as needed.

Appointments

Whether it's a visit to the doctor, a hairdresser's appointment or a booking for a back massage, try scheduling these from midday to late afternoon, when you know you'll be fully awake.

This will help you to, not only, process any important information, such as advice from your doctor, but to also make informed decisions: from the trivial, e.g., the exact length of your haircut to the more important, such as your healthcare plan.

It's important to note that if you're going to have any procedures or surgeries, the best time to have them is at the start of the physically-active phase of your day, which is usually from midday for night owls – i.e., categorically *not* in the first hour after waking, but at the very least 2 to 3 hours after the start of your natural rhythm's morning, but preferably later. This will ensure a speedy and more successful recovery. Even though the only studies that have proven this to work in practice were done on mice, it's plausible it translates to the best timing for humans to sustain an injury – which is basically what surgery is – as well.

Keep in mind that it's not only things as drastic as surgery; a simple manicure or teeth cleaning appointment, when scheduled at the right time it can save you from a nasty infection.

Going out

It's important to try and maintain your social life because, according to a 2017 study led by Christoph Randler, which examined over 4,500 people, evening types are a lot more likely to suffer from loneliness.

Now, there are rare individuals – like me – that revel in solitude; however, most people don't function well without a healthy social life. Having said that, please take the following into account:

If you have friends that love to organise tea parties early in the morning, talk to them and see if they wouldn't mind moving the time even just a little bit forward.

Also, remember that, according to Andrew Huberman, alcohol consumption will adversely affect the quality of your sleep. So, try to limit the amount of alcohol you consume when going out for drinks with your friends in the evening.

Attitudes

The night-owl syndrome is still regarded by many – including countless uninformed medical professionals – as a myth: a lifestyle gone wrong. And considering that for the longest time, society has idolised early risers, it may be challenging for those closest to you to understand or accept your new lifestyle changes – in spite of all the recently discovered scientific facts about the genetic makeup of night owls. For example, my Dad, an early bird, still tries to encourage me to go to bed earlier and worries about me. He says things like, 'You should sleep at night; staying up so late isn't good for you.' I just nod my head and smile. I know I'm not going to change his mind and that's ok.

Making the decision to stick to my guns has been the best thing I have ever done for my health and mental well-being, but I never expected that everyone in my life would agree with my choices. Thankfully, I have a loving husband who is not only very supportive but also a night owl himself.

I guess the best thing to do is to make peace with the fact that there will always be people around you who will shake their heads in disapproval. Your job isn't to change their minds but to ensure that you're looking after your well-being in the best way possible.

Exercise

Finally, I'm able to offer some good news to those of you unable to change your lifestyle, at least for now. If there's nothing you can do to change your work or school hours, there's one thing that you can introduce to your weekly regime that has been proven to either reduce the harmful effects of living out of alignment with your biological rhythm, and that's exercise.

A 2021 study analysed the data of over 380,000 individuals over an 11-year period. It found that those who engaged in regular exercise – either a minimum of 2.5h of moderate exercise or 75 min of intensive exercise per week – were able to either greatly decrease or almost eliminate their risk of dying of either cardiovascular disease or from cancer, despite poor sleep habits.

In addition, physical activity has been proven to improve the quality of sleep, not to mention that exercise aids in the production of melatonin, which helps with the onset of sleep.

All that is good and well; unfortunately, according to a recent study, an average night owl gets a lot less exercise than an average person. This is again attributed to trying to conform to an early riser's routine. Most night owls don't exercise in the morning, which is understandable because they want to get as much sleep as possible. What's unfortunate is that they don't exercise in the afternoon or evening either. Even though their energy levels are at an optimum by late afternoon/evening, night owls often don't exercise at that time because their evening social life routine doesn't typically accommodate for it.

However, if you happen to be one of the smart ones who regularly engages in physical activity, you should still try to do it at a time that best suits your chronotype. According to Matthew Walker, a good night's sleep that's in alignment with your natural rhythm lowers your blood pressure; this helps you get the best out of your physical activities and allows you to maintain a healthy heart.

Also, it might be a weird thing to say, but you should plan for getting injured. And, considering that the most likely time you might get injured is while you're active – particularly when you exercise – you should plan to be active in alignment with your circadian clock.

The science is clear on this: repair systems are more rapid and efficient during the active phase of your circadian cycle. In the case of night owls, this means anywhere from mid-afternoon to late evening. However, the most optimum window is between late afternoon to early evening. It's proven again and again that when owls try to exercise in the morning, it tends to make them tired rather than energised. It also means that if you do get injured in the morning, the healing process will be drawn out extensively.

Study

If you're a high school student, there aren't many options available to you that will allow you to navigate your night routine – unless your parents are willing to home-school you. However, in some countries, schools allow students to complete the last two years of high school (approximate age 16 to 18) via night school. But if you have to wake up in the morning, the only advice I can give you is to do everything you can to get as much as possible organised the night before. This means laying out your clothes ready for the morning, packing your school bag and preparing lunch the night before. You can also talk to your parents to see if it's possible to extend your waking time even by just 30 minutes. It might help to show them the data from the parenting section in chapter 6.

When it comes to higher education, there are plenty of options – at least in developed countries. The most obvious is studying online, although some higher education institutions offer on-campus night courses. I was in this position a few years ago when I tried to improve my writing skills; I enrolled with Open Universities Australia, which allowed me to study for my degree online – best decision I ever made!

Eating

When I told you my story at the start of the book, I didn't mention that aligning with my circadian rhythm was only partially responsible for my weight loss. I also incorporated time-restricted feeding into my routine – what you probably know as 'intermittent fasting'.

The latest research on intermittent fasting by world-renowned scholar and leading researcher on chronobiology Satchin Panda PhD shows that eating at the right time and limiting the hours when food is consumed offers vast benefits.

Some of the benefits of intermittent fasting include weight loss (for those who are overweight), prediabetes reversal, and effective management of type-2 diabetes. In addition, several months of consistent intermittent fasting improves kidney function, enhances immunity, reduces the risk of heart disease, and retrains your liver (and fat cells) to break down cholesterol and eradicate unwanted fat.

The above are some of the big and hairy things we really want to manage. But the more immediate benefits reported by people who have tried intermittent fasting for longer periods include better sleep, more energy during the day, and significantly less muscle and joint pain.

Other researchers echo Panda's advice; in fact, most of the scientific world today is in favour of intermittent fasting and recognises its many benefits. However, once again, the question of *when* to fast is a key factor in this practice.

Your metabolic rate is at its lowest during your biological night and most active about 12 hours after waking, during your biological afternoon-evening. The latest research suggests that we should eat only during the active phase of our cycle.

To gain the most benefits from this practice, you should start eating no earlier than an hour (or longer) after waking and stop eating at least 3 to 4 hours before bedtime. And if you have consumed a larger meal, you might need to allow 5 to 6 hours.

The reason why you shouldn't eat within the first hour of waking is that your body is still experiencing sleep inertia – slowed/reduced physical and cognitive performance – and isn't able to effectively process food at this time because the systems that deal with food consumption are just starting to fire up, slowly shifting from rest-and-restore phase to active phase. These systems include your microbiome, your stomach, systems responsible for the production of insulin and others.

***

Similarly, the body needs a food-free period in the evening to properly prepare you for sleeping. Abstaining from food for at least 3 to 4 hours before bedtime helps with the production of melatonin and the regulation of blood glucose.

To optimise your results, ensure that you eat the same number – regardless of whether you have 2 or 5 meals – at the same time each day. This really helps people who seem to always feel hungry – not just physically but emotionally. Eating at the same time each day (with no more than 30 minutes variance) helps the clock to plan for digestion and when to make you feel hungry, but more importantly, **it extends the time when you feel satiated.**

When I first decided I would not eat past 7:30 pm, it was really tough; I kept thinking about food. It took a few weeks of iron-clad willpower (although, I admit, there were plenty of hungry tears also) to stick to the cut-off time. But when I finally settled into the routine, the cravings and hunger disappeared – except once a month, when I get late night cravings for a day or two proceeding my period. Don't judge me, I'm human and despite best intentions, I usually succumb to my (very unhealthy) cravings during that window.

Overall, despite my cut-off time being 7:30 pm, I usually follow an 10:30 am to 7:00 pm eating window; Personally, I just feel better when I stop eating around 7:00 pm mostly because I'm usually able to fall asleep faster and easier if I stop eating earlier.

One of the main reasons why we need a break from food is that it activates *autophagy*. The easiest way to explain autophagy is, the body eats itself. But not in a gruesome or destructive way; quite the opposite, it consumes all the junk that has accumulated in your body, including old and damaged cells. It also uses the energy (glucose) that your body has stored up during the eating window, which helps you to maintain a healthy weight. It also breaks down and reuses old cell parts to help your body function more effectively.

Apart from its role in preventing and fighting disease, autophagy has recently been identified as playing a key role in the smooth running of your circadian rhythm because it regulates the liver clock and glucose metabolism.

Also, not incorporating autophagy into your daily schedule leads to an excessive build-up of the CRY1 gene – which suppresses the body's ability to draw on its glucose stores – and disrupts your circadian rhythm.

A disrupted rhythm reduces the abundance of the microbiota – the microorganisms living in the digestive tract that boost your metabolism, protect against bowel infections and help you maintain a healthy weight, among dozens of other things. Major research (in the last decade) shows that your microbiome can be easily reset by intermittent fasting.

Naps

Another interesting fact is that some people tend to function at their best when they implement napping into their routine. Even though napping is often enjoyed by people all over the world, the practice is more prevalent among warm-climate populations. It seems to be the body's natural way to deal with heat, forcing individuals out of the sun to avoid a heat stroke.

However, while naps help some people, they can diminish the quality of night sleep for others – particularly for the elderly, as some studies have shown.

Biphasic sleep

There's limited evidence which shows that some people perform best on a biphasic clock. According to investigative science journalist Zaria Gorvett, people used to call these *first sleep* and *second sleep*, which, some claim, used to be common in pre-industrial times. Biphasic means sleeping twice every night. The first sleep consists of only a couple of hours, followed by a break that lasts anywhere from a few minutes to several hours. Then the second sleep, which culminates the following morning. Biphasic sleep is a common phenomenon, although, through my interviews with everyday people, I found that, like the night owls, they feel it's something they need to fix. They expect to sleep through the night, with a solid 8-hour slumber. Thomas Wehr, a scientist, conducted a study to see if biphasic sleep is a natural part of life for some people. During the study, the subjects were deprived of alarm clocks, and as a result many naturally fell into a biphasic sleeping pattern.

These findings were confirmed by another scientist, David Samson. In 2015, he conducted a study among a remote community (that doesn't use electricity) in Madagascar. He asked them to wear activity trackers for ten days. The trackers revealed that most of the adults napped during the day and for many (49% of participants), the night consisted of an early, short phase sleep, followed by several hours of wakefulness and activity in the middle of the night, followed by another, longer phase of sleep. However, biphasic sleep is still a controversial concept in the chronobiology academic community as not enough research has been done to verify its validity and impact on health.

Environment

I hope you can see by now how important it is to protect your natural rhythm. However, I understand that in modern society, people are often limited, to varying degrees, in what they can do to align with their biological clock. But what you can't control about your lifestyle, you might make up for by controlling your environment.

For example, what **kind of lighting** do you have in your home? And **where is it positioned**?

During the day, ideally, you want as much natural light as possible flowing into the space you spend the most time. If you don't have that option, ensure that the ceiling lights are bright with a tone that mimics natural light. According to Samer Hattar PhD – an expert on light and circadian rhythms – exposure to plenty of light during the day is not only beneficial for maintaining your circadian rhythm in genetic alignment but also helps to lift your mood, improve learning and manage your appetite.

As soon as dusk arrives, switch off the ceiling lights and use lamps positioned as low as possible to the ground.

For example, on credenzas, side tables or even on the floor. Make sure that the tone of light is warm (yellow, orange, or even red) and that it's the dimmest light you can comfortably see in. Remember that once you switch from day light to evening light, it will take a few minutes for your retina to adjust, so try not to be tempted to switch to something brighter. This is important because bright lights in the evening and night are one of the biggest causes of circadian rhythm disruption – on par with the blue-light emitted by the screens on your devices, including your phone, laptop, TV etc.

Also, if you tend to wake up at night to use the toilet, position a couple of motion-activated, dim, red-coloured lights near the floor level. Red lights, as well as fireplaces and candlelight, are neutral and do not disrupt the sleep–wake cycle.

And if you want to check what time it is on your phone when you wake up in the middle of the night, make sure the phone brightness is set to the lowest setting and keep the phone turned away from your eyes (at an angle) so that you can still see the time, but the light isn't directly shining in your eyes.

Research shows that night owls are particularly sensitive to light, more so than any other chronotype. So be mindful of all the light in the evening and night in your environment. Samer Hattar says that you should do two things: reduce the brightness of your screens to the lowest possible setting – especially on TV (once again, waiting for your eyes to adjust) – and increase the warmth of the display.

Michelle Drerup PsyD of the Sleep Disorders Center says that keeping the room dark and its temperature between 10 and 15 degrees Celsius (60 and 67 F) is the best recipe for a good night's sleep – lights and too much temperature variance outside of this may result in disrupted sleep.

A noisy environment (e.g., if you live next to a railway line) is another reason why you might not feel rested when you wake up. You can reduce its impact by putting on some soothing music – white noise – at night to help you ride out any potential noise disruptions.

Finally, air pollution is an important factor in proper sleep hygiene and overall health. If you live in an area impacted by air pollution, it might pay to invest in an air filtration system at home and keep your windows closed at night.

Meditation

Some people find it hard to fall asleep, despite diligently following all of the advice mentioned in this book. If you are one of those people, you might want to try incorporating meditation or prayer into your routine. Even if you're not well versed in meditation or are not religious, something simple, such as taking a lavender-infused bath at night, is a powerful way to slow down your thoughts and prepare for bedtime.

Travel

The same study about loneliness I mentioned earlier in this chapter – in the section on 'Going out' – shows that late chronotypes are much more likely to show openness to new experiences; maybe that's why so many of the night owls I've met love to travel. And on that thought, I want to mention **jet lag**, which in some cases can be an advantage for night owls.

Depending on the time difference, morning larks often need at least two weeks to adjust their circadian rhythm to a new time zone in order to resume their morning routine and enjoy a full day of sight-seeing, whereas night owls are often able to enjoy all that the new location has to offer as soon as they land.

In my case, even though I'm always missing out on the many breakfast menus (that finish before 10:30 am) of beautiful cafes in my hometown, when I fly to Paris, I'm naturally up very early in the morning and can enjoy my holiday from day one. With my body clock still running on its previous setting, I get to join, albeit for a limited time, the early-riser society in all its glory and bask in the morning sun alongside the morning larks. Because I usually wake up around 9:30 am in my home town: Adelaide, Australia, which is 2:00 am in Europe, it means that when I arrive at my holiday destination, all I have to do is go to sleep around 3 hours later than my normal bedtime (which isn't too much of a struggle for me), and I'll be up around 5:00 am in e.g., Paris, giving me a slow morning, after which I can head out to a local cafe for brekky around 8:00 am – perfect! No jetlag, only minimal adjustment required – in that moment, I can experience life as a morning lark. I can enjoy this routine for about 1 to 2 weeks – before my circadian rhythm adjusts to the new light–dark cycle and I become a night owl again in my new location.

Illness

We all get sick sometimes. But it's when you are sick that alignment with your circadian rhythm is most critical. If, in all other instances, you're unable to follow your natural rhythm (because of work or study, for example), this is the one time you should call in sick and reset your rhythm – and try to get at least 8 hours of sleep.

Even though the study of chronobiology dates back to the 18th century, it's only in the last decade that we have discovered the clock's control over the immune system and its ability to respond to an attack.

According to Satchin Panda, there is no pill or medication in the world that can accelerate your recovery faster than getting the right amount of sleep that's aligned with your natural rhythm. That's because it is the only way to engage your immune response effectively. Also, the outcome of an illness is strongly connected to when you were initially exposed to the disease – whether it was viral, bacterial or parasitic. Your symptoms and length of the illness are greatly increased when the initial exposure took place during your rest phase.

This has great implications for night owls if the initial exposure to the illness occurred in the morning. If you're one of the many night owls who has a day job, you're likely to be engaging with potentially contagious co-workers. If you can limit close contact with others in the morning, when your body is still in the rest phase, you'll significantly reduce the symptoms and outcomes of many illnesses.

Asthma studies show reduced expression of genes responsible for optimum respiratory tract operation in adult patients with a misaligned circadian rhythm.

Finally, a disrupted clock is linked to increased cases of autoimmune diseases, such as multiple sclerosis, rheumatoid arthritis, Hashimoto thyroiditis and others. This is due to the prolonged neuroinflammation and demyelination, caused by the misaligned state.

Satchin Panda's lab has also recently discovered that the effectiveness of thousands of medications available on the market today could be significantly improved against a myriad of ailments if only taken at the **right** time of day – currently, there are over 100 medications that are officially recognised for their time-of-day efficacy. This is due to ongoing exciting research called chrono-pharmacology (or circadian medicine), which utilises timed administration of various drugs.

Some of the findings:

- Taking aspirin before bedtime, not in the morning, can half your risk of stroke,

- Giving cancer medication in the afternoon can make them twice as effective,

- Flu vaccinations given in the morning (for morning larks) produce more antibodies for older patients – I couldn't find info about this in relation to night owls.

Chapter Nine

Conclusion

If, like me, you are a night owl, I'd like to encourage you to rethink your lifestyle, your attitudes towards work, and your own internal monologue; and to understand that to live a healthy, productive and fulfilling life, you'll need to stop buying into this prevalent 'early-riser' religion.

If your job requires you to wake up early, it may be time to think about a career change or, at the very least, to discuss options with your employer to try and negotiate your working hours. From my own experience, adjusting my sleep schedule has been a priceless, life-changing experience.

And to everyone else, especially the people in charge of decisions that impact working hours, please reconsider the current working and school hours you have in place to take into account the health and productivity of the 70% of the population, which includes intermediates and night owls; you are putting their physical and mental health at risk by setting starting times so early in the morning. Why not consider different starting times for different employees? Adopt an attitude of flexibility. Encourage your employees and/or students to wake up naturally – without an alarm clock – and come to work in their own time. We don't know how many lives could be improved (and saved) by adopting such mentality. But even if you don't care about their health, imagine how such a change could reduce peak-hour traffic in major cities around the world.

I hope that we, as a society, might consider opening everything else a little later because, as it stands now, the world is skewed towards the 30% of the population: the early lark. Even most white-collar jobs start between 8 to 9 am, meaning that an average person has to wake up around 5 to 6 am to exercise, have a shower, eat and drive to work. If we could only delay work starting times to 10 or 11 am, the world would be a much happier and healthier place to live.

It isn't just the night owls and intermediates that suffer as a result of the current work and school starting times; there are plenty of morning larks working the night shift. All of this is causing an epidemic of physical and mental illness.

Remember that the best thing you can do for your circadian rhythm is to establish consistent, powerful anchors. A solid routine is the best way to ensure alignment and optimum operation of your biological clock and all the systems it controls. What you'll receive in return is health, wealth and (possibly) happiness – at least that's what I wish for you.

***

Thank you for reading my book; I hope I've been able to expand your knowledge about the circadian rhythm and the reality of being a night owl. If this book was useful to you, it would mean so much to me if you could post a review on whichever platform you prefer. Once again, thank you and remember, I'd love to hear about your personal experience and reflections – feel free to DM me on Twitter @sylviadziuba or Instagram (same handle).

About the Author

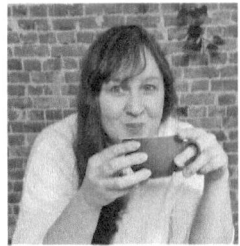

Sylvia Dziuba is an Australian author. She specialises in non-fiction genres, such as health, psychology, and culture. Using latest research, her writing offers unique perspectives on subjects with outdated opinions and biases.

If you'd like to learn more about any future books that she's working on, you can subscribe to her newsletter at sylviadziuba.com

You can also find her on social media – Twitter, Instagram and LinkedIn. Her handle is @sylviadziuba.

Below is a link to my YouTube channel:

youtube.com/@SylviaDziuba/

Acknowledgements

Firstly, I would like to thank the editor of this book, Heather Millar at Zest Communications, who did a fantastic job editing my manuscript. Also, a huge thank you to a very talented artist (who happens to be my daughter), Nell Dziuba, who illustrated the cover for this book.

But most importantly, I'd like to thank the researchers, scholars, investigative journalists and scientists that have made this book possible. Your papers, articles, research and studies have allowed me to delve headfirst into a deep examination of chronobiology and its relevance to night owls. Your research saves lives, emotionally and physically. I appreciate your ongoing exploration of and dedication to this field.

Please find below a list of professionals who were cited or consulted for this book in alphabetical order (by surname):

- Clare Anderson, Associate Professor at Monash University, Australia

- David Berson PhD, professor and chairman of neuroscience, Brown University, USA

- Sarah Chellappa PhD, a neuroscientist at the University of Cologne, Germany

- Prof Sean Drummond, clinical neuroscientist, Monash University, Australia

- Michelle Drerup PsyD of the Sleep Disorders Center, Cleveland Clinic, USA

- Dr Elise Facer-Childs, chronobiology & performance expert and researcher at Monash University, Australia

- Prof Russell Foster, world-renowned and award-winning chronobiologist, Sleep and Circadian Science Institute, Oxford University, UK

- Frederic Gachon, associate professor, physiology of circadian rhythms, Institute for Molecular Bioscience, The University of Queensland, Australia

- Zaria Gorvett, award-winning science journalist; Dr Carmel Harrington, author of The Sleep Diet

- Samer Hattar PhD, chief of the section on light and circadian rhythms at the National Institute of Mental Health, Bethesda, Maryland, USA

- Samuel Edward Jones, senior researcher, Institute for Molecular Medicine Finland

- Prof Guy Leschziner, Neurology & Sleep Medicine, King's College, London, UK

- Prof Laura Lewis, biomedical engineer, Boston University, USA

- Svetlana Maskevich, a psychologist and PhD candidate at Monash University, Australia

- Prof Sharon Naismith, neuropsychologist, University of Sydney, Australia

- Prof Satchin Panda PhD, scholar and researcher, a world-renowned expert on chronobiology

- Dr Gina Poe, neuroscientist, UCLA, USA

- Hans Reinke PhD, researcher, University of Duesseldorf, Germany

- Prof Kneginja Richter, University Clinic for Psychiatry and Psychotherapy, Paracelsus Medical University, Nuremberg, Germany

- Till Roenneberg PhD, professor of chronobiology, Institute of Medical Psychology, Ludwig-Maximilian University, Munich, Germany

- Prof David Samson PhD, researcher, University of Toronto, Mississauga, Canada

- Emmanuel Stamatakis, professor of physical activity, lifestyle and population health, University of Sydney, Australia

- Dr Caroline Sutton, researcher at Trinity College in Dublin, Ireland

- Prof Matthew Walker PhD, researcher and author of Why We Sleep, Neuroscience and Psychology,

University of California, Berkeley, USA

- Thomas Wehr, sleep scientist, National Institute of Mental Health, Bethesda, Maryland, USA.

www.ingramcontent.com/pod-product-compliance
Lightning Source LLC
Chambersburg PA
CBHW020325010526
44107CB00054B/1978